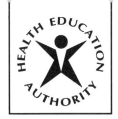

PROMOTING YOUNG PEOPLE'S SEXUAL HEALTH

A COMPENDIUM OF FAMILY PLANNING SERVICE PROVISION FOR YOUNG PEOPLE

Peter Aggleton
with Helen Chalmers, Susie Daniel and Ian Warwick

Developed by the Health Education Authority
and the Health & Education Research Unit
Institute of Education, University of London

Peter Aggleton is Professor in Education, Director of the Thomas Coram Research Unit and Co-Director of the Health and Education Research Unit at the Institute of Education, University of London.

Helen Chalmers and **Susie Daniel** are consultants working with the Health and Education Research Unit at the Institute of Education, University of London.

Ian Warwick is Assistant Director of the Health and Education Research Unit at the Institute of Education, University of London.

ACKNOWLEDGEMENTS

Anglia and Oxford
Dr Pat Troop, Regional Director of Public Health, Stephen Green, Health Policy Support Manager, Lori Brown, Kay Curtis, Dr Liz Greenhall, Dr Sue Halliday, Ms Joanna Hannam, Dr Tony Jewell, Ms Jo Jones, Dr Paul Loo, Dr Kate Nash, Dr Angela Owen-Smith, Ms Becky Pollard, Dr Maryan Pye, Justin Rolph, Dr Silas Sebugwawo, Dr Paul Scourfield, Dr Claire Smith.

Northern and Yorkshire
Prof. L Donaldson, Regional Director of Public Health, Dr Peter Hill, Deputy Director of Public Health, Paul Fallon, Head of Primary Care, Elaine Allen, Margaret Barnett, Liz Booth, Pam Dougal, Dr Janet Gallagher, Dr Charlotte Greg, Paul Hayton, June Hellon, Lesley Holt, Liz Hoyle, Jeanie Leggett, Dr Rosemary Livingstone, Margaret Millar, Nicola Power, Mike Ramsden, Lesley Richardson, Ian Robinson, David Russell, Sandi Scott, Iram Shar, Sandy Smart, Liz Smith, Chris Town, Gill Turner, Dr Linda Turner, Dr R D Walker, Cullagh Warnock, Kathy Waters, Dr Jan Wellbury, Janet Welsh.

North Thames
Dr Angela Jones, then Acting Regional Director of Public Health, Dr Jean Chapple, Consultant in Public Health Medicine, Danilo Armstrong, Dr Brenda Bean, Karen Bowden, Gina Burgess, Jackie Cahill, Justin Gaffney, Gill Heathcote, Dr Bela Reed, Dr Connie Smith.

North West
Prof. John Ashton, Regional Director of Public Health, Christine Owen, Health Policy and Development Coordinator, Dr Lesley Batchelor, Glynnis Francis, Dr Ellis Friedman, Liz Hall, Maureen Hollingbrooke, Alison Logan, Judi Noden, Trish Reid, Jean Rust, Sue Ryrie, Dr Phillada Shipp, Tim Smith.

South and West
Dr G Scally, Regional Director of Public Health, Dr Pauline Allen, Dr Elaine Cooper, Rosalie Gurr, Dr A Hill, Heather Litton, Alison Milchem, Ruth Milner-Scott, Pat Palmer, Dr Marianne Pitman, Dr Bill Poulson, Mrs Sandy Prior, Dr Sarah Randell, Jan Sanders, Sandra Stroffler, Linda Taylor, Dale Webb, Dr E White, Dr Brendan Yates.

South Thames
Dr Sue Atkinson, Regional Director of Public Health, Pat Dark, Senior Policy Advisor, Pat Bromage, Charlotte Dale, Billie Dawson, Dr Sylvia Elllis, John Harris, Mrs Janet Hoy, Neil Hunt, Dr Lois Lodge, Helen Massil, Jenny Oaks, Zoe Plant, Ann Richmond, Michael Rose, Linda Rossell, Doreen Rosser, Pauline Ruddy, Alison Rummey, Sue Ward, Dr Christine Watson, Maureen Willis.

Trent
Dr Lyndsey Davies, Regional Director of Public Health, Rae Magowan, Assistant Director of Public Health, Dr Jackie Abrahams, Dr E Butler, Janet Cozens, Dr Barbara Horton, Dr Ann Howard, Dr Sarah Hughes, Christine Humphries, Dr Sharon Jennings, Diana Marriott, Kate Moynihan, Hugh Nicolson, Mrs Gloria Percival, Ms Carol Power, Dr Greta Ross, Mr Henry Ruddock, Mrs Sheldon, Dr Tilzey, Dr Gill Wandless, Anne Ward, Dr Jenny Wordsworth.

West Midlands
Prof. Roy Griffiths, Regional Director of Public Health, Liz Biolik, Jill Campbell, Alice Cruttwell, Michelle Diaz, Jean Foster, Jo Jones, Terry Lawrence, Lucy Loveless, Ann Marie Morris, Rory Murray, Sarah New, Linda O'Sullivan, Dr Tony Robinson, Jenny Smith, Jo Smith.

Health Education Authority
Paul Lincoln, Business Team Director, Cathy Stillman-Lowe, Account Manager, Stuart Watson, Project Manager.

We would also like to thank members of the project reference group: Alison Hadley, Dr Aidan McFarlane, Margaret McGovern and Dr Tony Robinson. Margaret Jones of Brook Advisory Centres provided useful additional information.

Literature review undertaken by Peter Kelley; manuscript prepared by Gaby Critchley and Helen Thomas.

Names, addresses and service characteristics are correct at the time of writing, but are subject to alteration without notice. Future changes within the NHS may not be reflected at the time of going to press.

CONTENTS

Foreword   v

Introduction   1

Towards better practice   3

Service characteristics   6

REGIONAL LISTINGS

Anglia and Oxford
Young Person's Clinic, Haverill, and Walk-in Clinic, Bury St Edmunds   11
Newtown Health and Advice, Huntingdon, and The Place, St Neots   11
Bodywise, Kettering   12
Mancroft Advice Project, Norwich   14
Young Person's Clinic and Under 25s Clinic, Norwich   14
Family Planning Services, Oxford   15
Family Planning and Young Person Service – Youth Clinics, Peterborough   16

Northern and Yorkshire
The Pop Inn, Alnwick   18
Youth Counselling Service and Raffles Counselling Service, Carlisle   19
Young Person's Clinic, Gateshead   19
Hexham Young People's Centre, Hexham   20
Designated Young People's Clinics and The Men's Room, Leeds   21
Streetwise, Newcastle upon Tyne   22
Adolescent Clinics and Young People's Clinic, Ripon   24
The Grapevine, South Shields   25

North Thames
Family Planning Service, Queensway Health Centre, Hatfield   26
City and Hackney Young People's Services, London   26
KISS (Keep It Safe and Sexy), London Brook Advisory Service, London   28
Well Men's Service, London   28
Young People's Service, Harrow   29
Young Person's Health Advice Service, Romford and Barking   30

North West

Wirral Brook Advisory Centre, Birkenhead   32

Teenage Advisory Clinic, Bolton   33

Tameside Young People's Health Clinic and Peer Education Project,
    Denton   33

Merseyside Brook Advisory Centre, Liverpool   34

Young People's Family Planning Clinic, Macclesfield   35

The Youth Advice Shop, Warrington   36

South and West

The Junction Health Advisory Centre, Bournemouth   38

Young Adults' Drop-in Clinic, Burnham-on-Sea   38

Healthwise, Coleford Health Centre, Gloucester   39

Community Clinics for Young People, Southampton, Shirley, New Milton,
    Romsey and Thornhill   40

Sex Sense, Portsmouth   41

Cornwall Brook Advisory Centre, Redruth   42

Advisory Centre for Young People, Salisbury   43

South Thames

Youth Advisory Clinics, Bexleyheath, Blackfen and Erith   44

Young People's Drop-in Clinic, Brighton   45

Young Person's Clinic, Chatham   46

Sussed Sex in 'Number 18', Chichester   46

Family Planning Services for Young People, Optimum Health Services,
    London, and Brook-based services   47

Trent

Under 20s Clinic and Free Condom Clinics, Derby   49

Choices, Youth Clinic and Always, Doncaster   50

SHOP (Sexual Health Options Project), Ilkeston   51

Young People's Clinic, Leicester   52

Share Out (Seeking Health Advice, Reassurance and Education
    Open to Under 20s), Louth, Alford, Mablethorpe and Horncastle   53

Teenage Information Clinics and Teenage Sexual Health Clinic,
    Newark, Warsop, Kirkby, Sutton, Ollerton and Mansfield   54

Victoria Teenage Clinic, Nottingham   55

Sheffield Youth Clinic   56

West Midlands

Birmingham Brook Advisory Service, Birmingham   57

Just for You, Chelmsley Wood, Kingshurst and Solihull   58

Saturday Young People's Clinic, Hereford   59

Young People's Clinic, Longbridge   59

The Health Store, Nuneaton   60

Sexual Health Drop-in, Oldbury   61

Teen Clinic and Drop-in Clinic, Tipton   62

Young Person's Clinic, West Bromwich   63

Bibliography   64

Index   66

FOREWORD

If we are to achieve the 'Health of the Nation' targets on sexual health, it is important that every opportunity is taken to deliver services that are accessible and appropriate to people's needs. This compendium is an aid in planning and developing strategies for family planning for young people, and for purchasing family planning services. We are concerned that health promotion strategies are successful in adapting national targets for local situations, and that services are appropriate and effective.

The services outlined in this compendium bring together experiences in providing young people's family planning services from across England. The compendium's aim is to facilitate the exchange of information between professionals working in the field, and contribute to the development of these services.

The compendium should prove invaluable to purchasers and providers of family planning services. It contains detailed practical examples of service provision that should assist purchasers and providers aiming to maintain and develop useful interventions in providing family planning services for young people.

Promoting young people's sexual health is a meticulously researched and thoughtful piece of work, and its findings warrant equally careful and thoughtful consideration.

Tony Close
Chairman, Health Education Authority

INTRODUCTION

To be effective, family planning services for young people must be designed to meet their users' needs and be provided in an environment which is acceptable to young people. Although isolated examples of high-quality provision have been documented, there is little systematic information on services of this type. This compendium has been compiled by the Health Education Authority for purchasers and providers in an effort to bridge this gap.

The compendium aims to:

- illustrate the type of services that young people find most appropriate and are most likely to use
- enable professionals working in this field to contact each other and exchange information that will contribute to the development of these services
- encourage collaboration between specialist family planning services and other statutory and voluntary agencies working with young people.

The compendium provides a region-by-region listing of selected family planning services for young people, describing the range of services on offer, the setting in which these services are provided, and the ways in which the services are designed to appeal to their users.

All the organisations listed are willing to provide further information about their work, and each entry therefore includes details of how to contact the organisation. The section entitled 'Towards better practice' summarises the issues that need to be taken into account when setting up or developing sexual and reproductive health services for young people.

It should be noted that this is by no means an exhaustive list of all work with young people, nor is it a comparative description of service provision within or between regions. Only agencies offering contraceptive services and nominated through each region's Director of Public Health are included in the compendium. Exclusion of a particular agency does not imply that its services are not of a high standard. Many centres offering excellent advice or referral services, for example, could not be included.

TOWARDS BETTER PRACTICE

The services described in this compendium highlight a number of issues that need to be taken into account when setting up new family planning and sexual health services for young people or when developing existing ones. This chapter summarises these considerations and offers guidance on what has worked in practice. Although it will be particularly useful to those involved in establishing new services, it may also serve as a checklist against which to evaluate aspects of existing provision. Supporting examples from the compendium are given at the end of the chapter.

Service settings

So that young people can feel at ease with a service appropriate to their needs, family planning and sexual health services should be made available to them in a variety of settings. Young people should be able to access services via:

- specialist clinics;
- GPs;
- youth advisory services;
- community-based outreach work.

Range of services

A wide range of family planning and sexual health services should be available so that services are appropriate to individual needs, including:

- a full range of condoms, including extra-strong and female condoms;
- emergency contraception;
- dual methods of contraception, in order to offer protection against STDs as well as pregnancy;
- smear tests;

- on-the-spot pregnancy tests;
- STD tests, including on-the-spot testing and HIV-related counselling;
- referral to STD services;
- advice and referral for termination of pregnancy;
- advice and counselling on the full range of sexual issues likely to affect young people, with referral as necessary.

Service integration

In order to offer a coherent approach to the promotion of young people's sexual and reproductive health, efforts should be made to integrate the various aspects of service provision. This means bringing together services for the prevention and treatment of STDs including HIV, services linked to contraceptive provision and advice, and services concerned with the promotion of more general aspects of young people's health.

Accessibility

Easy access is important if family planning services are to be widely available to young people. This can be achieved by:

- basing services in, or close to, schools, colleges and youth centres;
- basing services in shopping centres, arcades and other places where young people meet;
- making sure that services are close to public transport and provide disabled access;
- making sure that services are open at times when young people can use them, e.g. after school, in the early evening and at weekends;
- encouraging young men to attend by providing separate services for them, such as young men's clinics;
- advertising services widely and in ways that will reach young people, such as through local radio, GP services and the local grapevine;
- signposting services in ways that young people find appropriate.

Atmosphere and image

The environment in which services are provided should appeal to young people, particularly by avoiding the 'clinical' atmosphere often associated with hospitals and hospital-based care. The views of potential service users can be canvassed in schools and youth centres through small-scale surveys or group discussions. While there are no hard-and-fast rules to follow, ways of creating an appropriate atmosphere can include:

- decorating waiting areas with posters and health promotion materials designed for young people;
- providing waiting areas with young people's magazines;
- making refreshments available;
- installing music, television and videos;
- arranging seating in waiting areas informally;
- asking staff to wear everyday clothes.

Staff selection and training

Staff should be specially chosen for their interest in, and commitment to, working with young people. To be most effective, staff may need training on issues linked to:

- approachability;
- developing a non-judgemental attitude;
- communication skills, with particular regard to discussing sexual matters;
- reassuring users on the issue of confidentiality;
- awareness of equal opportunities, to ensure that services are made equally available to 'non-traditional' service users, including young heterosexual men, young lesbians and gay men, young disabled people, young people with learning difficulties and young people from minority ethnic communities.

A number of the services in this compendium have initiated training programmes for their staff.

Monitoring and evaluation

In order to be accessible and appropriate to young people, and in order to maintain their effectiveness, services require careful monitoring and evaluation. This can be carried out in a variety of ways, including:

- initial and ongoing assessments of young people's needs;
- monitoring of service-user characteristics;
- monitoring of service appropriateness and acceptability;
- evaluating the effects of service provision locally.

In the space available here we can point to only some of the important considerations to take into account when planning or developing family planning and sexual health services for young people. Further guidance can be found in the *Key Area Handbook HIV/AIDS and Sexual Health*,

Service Characteristics

	SC	GP	YAS	CBW	YM	INT	ST	PAGE
Anglia & Oxford								
YP's Clinic (Haverhill)	●							11
Walk-In Clinic (Bury St Edmunds)	●							11
Newtown Health and Advice (Huntingdon)	●							11
The Place (St Neots)	●							11
Bodywise (Kettering)	●			●		●	●	12
Mancroft Advice Project (Norwich)	●		●			●		14
YP's Clinic (Norwich)	●							14
Under 25s Clinic (Norwich)	●							14
Family Planning Services (Oxford)	●				●		●	15
Family Planning and YP's Service – Youth Clinics (Peterborough)	●		●	●		●	●	16
Northern & Yorkshire								
The Pop Inn (Alnwick)	●			●		●		18
Youth Counselling Service (Carlisle)	●		●					19
Raffles Counselling Service (Carlisle)	●		●					19
YP's Clinic (Gateshead)	●				●	●		19
Hexham's YP's Centre (Hexham)	●			●		●		20
Designated YP's Clinics (Leeds)	●		●			●		21
The Men's Room (Leeds)	●		●			●		21
Streetwise (Newcastle-u-Tyne)	●		●	●		●	●	22
Adolescent Clinics (Ripon)	●	●	●			●	●	24
YP's Clinic (Ripon)	●	●	●	●		●	●	24
The Grapevine (South Shields)	●		●			●		25
North Thames								
Family Planning Service (Hatfield)	●			●			●	26
City & Hackney YP's Services (London)	●			●	●	●		26
KISS London Brook Advisory Service	●							28
Well Men's Service (London)					●			28
YP's Service (Harrow)	●		●	●			●	29
YP's Health Advice Service (Romford & Barking)	●			●				30
North West								
Wirral Brook Advisory Centre (Birkenhead)	●	●	●	●		●	●	32
Teenage Advisory Clinic (Bolton)	●							33
Tameside YP's Health Clinic & Peer Education Project (Denton)	●		●	●		●	●	33
Merseyside Brook Advisory Centre (Liverpool)	●							34
YP's Family Planning Clinic (Macclesfield)	●							35
The Youth Advice Shop (Warrington)	●		●					36

SC = specialist clinics   GP = general practitioners   YAS = youth advisory services   CBW = community-based outreach wor[k]

	SC	GP	YAS	CBW	YM	INT	ST	PAGE
South & West								
The Junction Health Advisory Centre (Bournemouth)	●		●					38
Young Adults' Drop-in Clinic (Burnham-on-Sea)	●	●						38
Healthwise (Gloucester)	●		●				●	39
Community Clinics for YP (Southampton, Shirley, New Milton, Romsey and Thornhill)	●			●				40
Sex Sense (Portsmouth)	●		●	●			●	41
Cornwall Brook Advisory Centre (Redruth)	●							42
Advisory Centre for Young People (Salisbury)	●		●			●		43
South Thames								
Youth Advisory Clinics (Bexleyheath, Blackfen and Erith)	●							44
YP's Drop-in Clinic (Brighton)	●			●			●	45
YP's Clinic (Chatham)	●							46
Sussed Sex in 'Number 18' (Chichester)	●		●					46
Family Planning Services for YP (Deptford)	●		●					47
Optimum Health Services (London)	●		●					47
Trent								
Under 20s Clinic (Derby)	●		●			●		49
Free Condom Clinics (Derby)	●		●					49
Choices (Doncaster)	●		●		●		●	50
Youth Clinic (Doncaster)	●		●	●	●			50
Always (Doncaster)	●	●	●	●	●			50
HOP (Ilkeston)	●		●	●		●		51
YP's Clinic (Leicester)	●		●				●	52
Share Out (Louth, Alford, Mablethorpe and Horncastle)	●		●	●	●	●		53
Teenage Info Clinics and Teenage Sexual Health Clinic (Newark, Warsop, Kirkby, Sutton, Ollerton and Mansfield)	●							54
Victoria Teenage Clinic (Nottingham)	●						●	55
Sheffield Youth Clinic	●		●	●		●	●	56
West Midlands								
Birmingham Brook Advisory Service	●			●	●	●	●	57
Just for You (Chelmsley Wood, Kingshurst and Solihull)	●						●	58
Saturday YP's Clinic (Hereford)	●		●			●		59
YP's Clinic (Longbridge)	●							59
The Health Store (Nuneaton)	●		●	●		●		60
Sexual Health Drop-in (Oldbury)	●			●		●	●	61
Teen Clinic (Tipton)	●	●						62
Drop-in Clinic (Tipton)	●	●						62
YP's Clinic (West Bromwich)	●	●						63

YM = specially dedicated services for young men   INT = integrated services   ST = training for own staff

published by the Department of Health in 1993, and in many of the other
publications listed in the bibliography at the end of this compendium.

In order to help you use this compendium more effectively, you may find it
helpful to refer to the table on pages 6-7 which offers an at-a-glance guide
to different organisations. It is arranged regionally and by type of service.
That way, you can find local services of the kind in which you are interested.
For example, if you are a GP thinking about setting up a service, you may
want to know where other GPs are providing such a service. Or you may
be thinking about initiating a staff training programme, and be looking for
somewhere with established training. The table provides easy access to
where in the compendium you might find further information about such
a service. It has been developed to help you find particular services and is
not intended to offer a comparison between services. Moreover, there is no
suggestion that organisations providing more services are better than those
providing fewer. When using this compendium, please remember that
service development is occurring all the time, so the information you will
find here should be taken as a guide to what is currently available.

REGIONAL LISTINGS

Young Person's Clinic, Haverill, and Walk-In Clinic, Bury St Edmunds

■ **Setting**
Suburban with rural catchment. Health centres.

■ **Principal aims and objectives**
To provide a confidential contraceptive and information service.

■ **Services offered**
Staffing. 1 physician, 1 nurse, 1/2 receptionists.

Advice/counselling. By medical and nursing staff. Referral for psychosexual counselling.

Contraception/sexual-health services. Oral contraception, condoms (extra-strong available), implant, cap/diaphragm, after-sex emergency contraception. Smear tests. On-the-spot pregnancy testing. Referral for termination of pregnancy. STD testing referred to GUM services.

Outreach via roadshows, health-day displays.

Telephone helpline.

■ **Appropriateness and acceptability**
Advertising via leaflets and booklet. Health shops promote service.

Service open Thursday early evening, Saturday mid-morning. Disabled access. Drinks machine. Health promotion carried out.

Written policy on confidentiality. Statement on all publicity.

Good links with health promotion and GUM services. Links with Suffolk Sexual Health Focus Group.

■ **Evaluation**
Patient satisfaction survey (not solely for young people). Suggestions boxes. Korner.

■ **Contact**
Dr Claire Smith
Consultant, Family Planning
  and Reproductive Health Care
Bloomfield House Health Care
Looms Lane
Bury St Edmunds
Suffolk IP33 1HE

Tel: 01284 763401
Fax: 01284 724374

Written enquiries preferred.

Newtown Health and Advice, Huntingdon, and The Place, St Neots

■ **Setting**
Towns. Clinics.

Principal aims and objectives
To provide a comprehensive service to young people including family planning, pregnancy testing and support. To provide increased

provision of counselling aimed towards the promotion of healthy lives for young people. To provide a broader service than family planning and to develop it in response to what young people identify as their needs.

■ Services offered
Staffing. 1 physician, 2 family planning trained nurses, 1 coordinator, 1 male clinical nurse specialist (HIV).

Advice/counselling. Nurse/doctor provides pre- and post-termination of pregnancy counselling, plus can refer to specialist counsellor at hospital. Direct access to voluntary young people's counselling service in Huntingdon, which provides broad-based youth counselling.

Contraception/sexual-health services. Wide range including condoms, strong condoms, lubricant. On-the-spot pregnancy testing. Referral for termination of pregnancy. Smear testing. Refer to GUM services for STD testing and HIV counselling and testing. One clinic doctor works in GUM.

Information advice line with clinic information and advice on emergency contraception access.

Work in schools and colleges. Work with local health promotion service.

■ Appropriateness and accessibility
Service developed in response to survey of young people's needs.

Service advertised by posters, leaflets and cards developed jointly with young people. Distributed widely to youth venues.

Consultations by drop-in sessions with follow-up appointments.

Dedicated space for young people's clinic at The Place. Sessions held late Monday and Thursday afternoons.

Disabled access.

Music, videos. Drinks available.

Policy on confidentiality displayed on all posters and discussed at first visit.

Good links with schools, social services, youth services, psychology, health promotion, school nurses, learning disability services. Local schools include clinic information in teacher induction pack. Open evening for local people and parents about services.

■ Evaluation
Use Community Information System which barcodes all clinic activities. Report available for 1994–5.

Young people on management committee provide feedback from their groups. Occasional questionnaires to young people.

■ Contact
Dr Angela Owen-Smith
Clinical Manager, Children's Services
Primrose Lane
Huntingdon
Cambridgeshire PE18 6SE

Tel: 01480 415211
Fax: 01480 415212

Telephone or written enquiries. Visits by arrangement.

Bodywise, Kettering
(Health advice for under 25s)

■ Setting
Town with rural surroundings. Health clinics and local colleges.

■ Principal aims and objectives
To provide a health service that specifically addresses the needs of young people aged 13–25 years. To work jointly with local youth

services. To enable young people to make informed decisions about their lifestyle, and to enable them to recognise and control risks affecting their health.

■ Services offered

Staffing. Bodywise team coordinator, assistant coordinator, 2 nurses, 1 administrator and clerical support. Clinic staff: 1 health adviser/nurse, 1 physician, 1 male counsellor or 1 male youth worker, occasionally 1 receptionist/clerk.

Advice/counselling. Within drop-in sessions by a counselling qualified youth worker. Counsel on any issue and provide ongoing support.

Contraception/sexual health care services. Full contraceptive service including a range of condoms. On-the-spot pregnancy testing. After-sex emergency contraception. Referral to British Pregnancy Advisory Service or via GP for termination of pregnancy. Referral to GUM services for STDs. Do pre- and post-test HIV counselling.

Outreach. To youth clubs and uniformed organisations on health and sexual health. Work with Young Carers group. Work with multi-disciplinary team for sex offenders. Sexual-health work with young people with disabilities.

Development of resources. Looklet booklet for young people. *Parents' guide to teens/Teens' guide to parents.*

Bodywise van and trailer, with coffee bar, television/video, radio and health leaflets/posters. Links with detached youth workers. Staffed by nurse (family planning), addictions outreach worker and a youth worker. Always at least one male and one female staff.

Fortnightly 'agony aunt' column in local newspaper by Bodywise staff.

■ Appropriateness and accessibility

Located in local health centres, drugs services and colleges.

Lunchtime sessions at colleges. Three Monday sessions – one midday and two late afternoon/evening. One Saturday midday session.

Easy access, with music, drinks.

Clinical links to GUM services, HIV workers, dietary services, and addiction services. Alliances with youth services, counselling agencies, Lions Clubs and a range of multi-agency forums.

Clear written confidentiality policy, communicated to young people at first visit.

Advertised through colleges, street work, youth clubs and churches with leaflets, cards and posters.

Bodywise information telephone line available five days a week, plus contraceptive advice line seven days a week.

■ Evaluation

Occasional audits. Evaluation of van/trailer. Suggestions box. Client-led discussions. Korner.

■ Contact

Lori Brown
Bodywise Coordinator
Oakwood House
St Mary's Hospital
London Road
Kettering NN15 7PW

Tel: 01536 493233
Fax: 01536 493250

Written or telephone enquiries.

Mancroft Advice Project, Norwich

■ Setting
Urban/suburban. Youth advisory project.

■ Principal aims and objectives
To offer free and confidential information, advice and counselling to young people aged 25 and under in Norwich and the surrounding area.

■ Services offered
Staffing. 1 project coordinator, 7 counsellors, 5 youth workers.

Advice/counselling. Crisis, one-off and ongoing counselling by qualified counsellors. Advocacy service in relation to Children Act Assessments, DSS support and visits to GUM services and family planning services.

Contraception/sexual-health services. Pregnancy tests on a drop-in basis. Referral to Norwich family planning service or GP service for all other contraceptive needs.

Support groups for young fathers, young mothers, sexual abuse survivors, young pregnant women.

■ Appropriateness and accessibility
Focused advertising in clubs, public houses and on streets.

Purpose-built youth centre in city centre location. Youth centre has coffee bar, computers, information database, childcare space and equipment, disabled access, large range of leaflets, posters and other resources.

Drop-in and appointment system. Service offered Monday–Friday early afternoon to early evening.

Counselling appointments can be made outside these hours.

Clear confidentiality policy.

Links with Health Information Shop, Women's Health Information Service, Gay Men's Health Project, drug counselling agencies.

■ Evaluation
Monitoring of numbers of young people using service, pregnancy tests and results, referrals, leaflets taken.

Two young people on the management committee provide user feedback. Young people's forum open to all young people and report sent to management committee.

Developing evaluation of counselling.

■ Contact
Justin Rolph
Coordinator
The Risebrow Centre
Chantry Road
Norwich NR2 1QZ

Tel: 01603 766994

Telephone contact preferred.

Young Person's Clinic and Under 25s Clinic, Norwich

■ Setting
Town with rural feeder areas. Health clinic.

■ Principal aims and objectives
To provide young people with a comprehensive and confidential family planning service.

■ Services offered
Staffing. 1 physician, 1 nurse, 1 receptionist per session.

Advice/counselling. Related to family planning and pre- and post-termination of pregnancy. Pyschosexual counselling provided by trained staff.

Contraception/sexual-health services. Condoms and other contraceptive services, including dual method. On-the-spot pregnancy tests. Referral for termination of pregnancy. After-sex emergency contraception. Smear tests. Refer to GUM services for STD-related concerns.

Some domiciliary visits if necessary.

Limited work in schools by family planning nurses.

■ Appropriateness and accessibility

Initial poster/media campaign linked to the launch of the service. Information available in libraries, schools and youth clubs.

Consultations offered on a drop-in basis one day a week, including the early evening and Saturday mornings.

Relatively informal atmosphere including music and informal staff clothing.

Close to city centre, 100 yards from bus station and close to local college.

■ Evaluation

Initial service user profile. Suggestions book. Waiting-time survey. Korner.

■ Contact

Dr Kate Nash
Principal Medical Officer
Central Family Planning Clinic
2–4 Brunswick Road
Norwich NR2 2HA

Tel: 01603 287345
Fax: 01603 287358

Written or telephone enquiries. No visits.

Family Planning Services, Oxford

■ Setting

Urban. Family planning centre in health clinic.

■ Principal aims and objectives

To enable people to enjoy the sexual activity of their choice without causing harm to themselves or others. To provide clinical contraceptive care. To provide training and advice to primary health-care workers. To educate other health care professionals. To provide family planning information to the general public.

■ Services offered

Staffing. 1–2 physicians, 1–2 nurses, 1 receptionist/clerk. Between sessions, nurse is available to issue repeat prescriptions and emergency contraception.

Advice/counselling. Psychosexual counselling, pre-conception care/advice, general gynaecological advice, termination of pregnancy service has counsellor for pre- and post-counselling. For broader issues refer to youth counselling services.

Contraception/sexual-health services. Wide range of contraceptive services including condoms, strong condoms, lubricant, female condoms. On-the-spot pregnancy testing. Referral for termination of pregnancy. Smear tests. Some STD testing. Refer most STDs to GUM services.

Outreach by clinic doctor, including training of youth workers and visits to youth clubs. Employ a sexual health advisory teacher (75% health authority, 25% LEA) to work in schools and with teachers. Visits to clinic as part of personal and social education programmes.

Phoneline available during opening hours.

■ Appropriateness and accessibility

Services advertised in the telephone directory and occasionally in the local newspaper.

Wide distribution of leaflets to chemists, GPs, libraries, Citizens' Advice Bureaux, schools, youth clubs.

Information available on Regional Health Information Line and via the County Council Information Terminal.

Consultations offered on drop-in and appointment basis.

Sessions six days a week at central clinic and at varying times of week in 11 other centres throughout the area.

Mainly Men Clinic one evening each week staffed by men and providing individual consultations – not specific to young men.

Clear code of confidentiality. Training for all reception staff and discussed regularly at staff meetings.

Easy access to dedicated clinic.

Television.

Links to GUM services, youth services, local education authority, health promotion, GPs, children's homes, mother and baby home, and school nurses. Joint training with GPs and GUM staff. Member of range of multi-disciplinary and multi-agency forums.

■ Evaluation

Service user satisfaction survey. Korner with additional information.

■ Contact

Dr Liz Greenhall
Director, Family Planning Services
Alec Turnbull Clinic
East Oxford Health Centre
Cowley Road
Oxford OX4 1XD

Tel: 01865 798196
Fax: 01865 204411

Written or telephone enquiries.

Family Planning and Young Person Service – Youth Clinics, Peterborough

■ Setting

Town with rural feeder areas. Health centres/schools/colleges.

■ Principal aims and objectives

To provide young people with confidential contraceptive advice and resources. To provide young people with confidential advice on sexual health issues.

Services offered

Staffing. 1 physician, 2 nurses, 2 receptionists per session (Saturday clinic), 3 nurses (Monday clinic).

Advice/counselling. Provided on a range of issues relating to sexual and reproductive health, including choice of contraception. HIV testing and counselling (staff trained by National AIDS Counselling Training Unit). Will accompany young person if referred to GUM services.

Contraceptive/sexual-health services. Wide range of contraceptive services including condoms and dual method. On-the-spot pregnancy tests. Referral for termination of pregnancy to GP or British Pregnancy Advisory Service.

After-sex emergency contraception. Smear tests. Outreach work in colleges, schools, youth clubs and probation service.

Displays at local events such as health fairs and health days at school.

Helpline being set up.

■ Appropriateness and accessibility

Service advertised via posters/leaflets, local radio/press, health fairs, clubs/pubs/entertainment places, libraries, health promotion service and outreach workers. Also by word of mouth.

Specially appointed reception staff to enhance welcoming atmosphere.

Drop-in and appointment service. Specialist young people's service available one evening a week and Saturday morning with additional local clinics throughout North West Anglia Health Care Trust.

Good public transport access. Clear statement of confidentiality.

Good links with local HIV/AIDS projects, local AIDS action group, Drink Sense, community drug service, probation services, women's centre, health promotion service, GUM services, schools and children's homes.

■ Evaluation
Service user questionnaires. Korner.

■ Contact
Kay Curtis
Family Planning, Young Person's Coordinator
City Health Clinic
Wellington Street
Peterborough PE1 5DU

Tel: 01733 312931
Fax: 01733 555763

Telephone contact preferred, Monday–Thursday mornings.

The Pop Inn, Alnwick

■ Setting
Town with large rural catchment area.
In community centre near
to secondary school.

■ Principal aims and objectives
To encourage a multi-disciplinary
approach to the meeting of young
people's health needs. To assist
in the promotion of the health triangle:
physical, emotional, mental. To educate
young people to be responsible for
their own health, e.g. risks of smoking,
alcohol consumption, poor nutrition,
casual relationships. To provide a
confidential listening ear. To reduce
the incidence of teenage pregnancy
as required in Health of the Nation
targets. To make young people aware
of the risks of STDs and encourage
them to take steps to avoid them. To
link young people to the appropriate
sources of help.

■ Services offered
Staffing. 1 family planning doctor,
1 school nurse, 1 community worker,
school medical officer twice a month,
physiotherapist twice a month,
HIV/AIDS charge nurse once a
month.

Advice/counselling. Provided by nurse
and doctor.

Contraceptive/sexual-health services.
A wide range of contraceptive services
including condoms, strong condoms.
On-the-spot pregnancy testing.

Clinical testing referred to GUM
services.

Group work for smoking cessation and
alcohol misuse.

Work in youth clubs and other
schools.

■ Appropriateness and accessibility
Services are advertised in the local
newspaper. Posters and leaflets in
schools, baths, sports centres, shops
and weekly school bulletin, *What's on.*

Consultations offered on drop-in
basis.

Sessions offered at community centre
one lunchtime each week at a
dedicated time.

Drinks and healthy snacks available.
Pool, table tennis, television and video,
music and magazines during session.

Confidentiality advertised on posters
and discussed at first visit.

Easy access from local school.

Links to schools, community centre
and residential children's home.

■ Evaluation
Evaluation of service user numbers,
user satisfaction, ages, service accessed
and gender. Korner.

■ Contact
Mrs Jeannie Leggett
Locality Manager
Bondgate Clinic
Infirmary Drive

Alnwick
Northumberland NE66 2NS

Tel: 01665 602661
Fax: 01665 510581

Written or telephone enquiries
welcome. Visits out of session times.

Youth Counselling Service and Raffles Counselling Service, Carlisle

■ **Setting**
Urban.

Principal aims and objectives
To reduce the number of teenage
pregnancies. To support young people
in safer sex and personal relationships.
To promote safer sex. To promote
harm reduction among drug users.

■ **Services offered**
Staffing. Youth Counselling Service:
1 physician, 2 nurses, 1 receptionist/
clerk. Raffles Counselling Service:
2 family planning nurses, 1 nurse
trained in drugs-related issues,
1 youth worker.

Advice/counselling. Provided by nurses
and doctor.

Contraception/sexual-health services.
Wide range of contraceptive services
including condoms and strong
condoms. On-the-spot pregnancy
testing. Referral for termination of
pregnancy. Smear tests. Referral for
HIV and most STD testing to GUM
services.

Helpline available via family planning
services number during office hours.

■ **Appropriateness and accessibility**
Services advertised in the local
telephone directory. Leaflets and
posters distributed to schools.

Consultations offered on drop-in and
appointment basis.

Sessions offered at Youth Counselling
Service Monday midday and
Thursday late afternoon. Sessions at
Raffles Counselling Service one
afternoon each week.

Confidentiality a priority.

Easy access to both sites.

Links to principal health promotion
officer/district HIV officer and some
young people's services.

■ **Evaluation**
Questionnaires. Suggestions box.
Korner.

■ **Contact**
Mrs Liz Hoyle/Ms June Hellon
Locality Manager/Senior Clinical
  Nurse
Central Clinic
50 Victoria Place
Carlisle CA1 1HN

Tel: 01228 36451
Fax: 01228 515610

Written or telephone enquiries.

Young Person's Clinic, Gateshead

■ **Setting**
Urban. Health centre.

■ **Principal aims and objectives**
To provide a confidential service to
young people, with easy access and a
comprehensive sexual-health service,
including the giving of advice and
information. To provide sessions with
appropriately trained staff, at
convenient times and in a convenient
location.

■ Services offered
Staffing. 1 physician, 2 nurses (including nurse who runs sex education in local schools), 1 receptionist/clerk.

Advice/counselling. Provided mainly by doctor and nurse, about psychosexual needs, periods, saying 'no', safer sex and other issues. Referral as necessary.

Contraceptive/sexual-health services. A wide range of contraceptive services including condoms and strong condoms. On-the-spot pregnancy testing and direct referral to hospital for termination of pregnancy. No implants at sessions. Smear tests and chlamydia tests available. All other STDs referred to GUM services.

Out of office hours, recorded message service with information about next clinic sessions for emergency contraception. Staff available during office hours.

Outreach by health trust community development workers and the family planning domiciliary nurse to promote the clinic sessions.

■ Appropriateness and accessibility
Services are advertised in the local phone book and occasionally in the newspaper. Publicity is distributed via schools and colleges, World AIDS Day activities and individual staff.

Consultations offered on drop-in basis.

Sessions offered at health centre one late afternoon each week.

Signposting to clinic session, and health videos and posters in clinic area.

Confidentiality discussed with young person at first visit and documentation provided on the issue. Good public transport available to clinic.

Links to GUM services, psychology services, termination of pregnancy services (NHS and private) and community education. Medical officer on various sub-groups and clinical service development groups. Have a local sex education resource group headed by health promotion officer for young people.

■ Evaluation
Survey of young people's likes and dislikes about service.

■ Contact
Dr Lynda Turner/Lesley Holt
Family Planning Manager/Family
  Planning Coordinator
Gateshead Healthcare Trust
  Headquarters
Whinney House
Durham Road
Low Fell
Gateshead NE9 5AR

Tel: 0191 402 6012
Fax: 0191 402 6001

Written or telephone enquiries welcome. Visits out of session times.

Hexham Young People's Centre, Hexham

■ Setting
Rural town with large rural catchment area. Community centre.

■ Principal aims and objectives
To provide access to appropriate services for young people regarding sexual health and counselling. To make the service broader than family planning, and to provide it within a young people's environment that is user-friendly. To ensure anonymity for young people and guarantee that they see the same staff, for continuity of care.

■ Services offered

Staffing. 1 physician, 1 family planning/school nurse, 1 youth worker, 1 youth worker as receptionist/clerk, occasionally 2 health promotion officers and another youth worker.

Advice/counselling. Provided by trained youth worker and doctor. Developing links with local mental health services. Developing peer counselling.

Contraception/sexual-health services. Wide range of contraceptive services including condoms and strong condoms. On-the-spot pregnancy testing. Referral for termination of pregnancy. Smear tests. Referral for HIV counselling and tests.

Taster sessions (group work) on sex, drugs, stopping smoking, self-defence for young women, mental health/self-awareness. Eight-week smoking cessation course.

Work in local schools, including two schools for children with special needs. Work with primary health care teams, school nurses, teachers, mental health care providers and voluntary groups.

■ Appropriateness and accessibility

Services advertised by clinic doctor speaking to all school assemblies in the area. Newspaper articles and radio advertisements/interviews. Leaflets and posters distributed widely to libraries, youth clubs, Citizens' Advice Bureaux.

Consultations offered on drop-in basis. Appointments for follow-up.

Sessions offered at community centre one afternoon each week at dedicated time.

Drinks and snacks available. Music and health promotion information.

Confidentiality discussed at first visit. Advertised on all publicity.

Good access from schools and town centre.

Links to education service, voluntary organisations (housing, young women's group), GPs, school health services, PTA/governors, child health services, psychology service. Involved in network of young people's health centres and other multi-disciplinary forums.

Young people's steering group is supported by youth worker(s). Feeds information into multi-disciplinary steering group.

■ Evaluation

Comments board. Korner with fuller details.

■ Contact

Dr Gill Turner
Northumberland Child Health Centre
John Street
Ashington NE63 0SE

Tel: 01670 856185
Fax: 01670 856144

Written or telephone enquiries.

Designated Young People's Clinics and The Men's Room, Leeds

■ Setting

Urban. Health centres.

■ Principal aims and objectives

To address issues of unplanned pregnancy and HIV/STDs by making young people aware of the services available and providing counselling. To offer a free drop-in confidential service.

■ Services offered
Staffing. 2 physicians, 2 nurses and
1 receptionist/clerk in each of the three
Young People's Clinics. 1 male nurse at
The Men's Room, 1 receptionist/clerk.

Advice/counselling. Provided by
nurses/doctors. All staff completed
HIV basic counselling course.
Referral for termination of pregnancy
counselling.

Contraception/sexual-health services.
Wide range including strong condoms
and dual method. On-the-spot
pregnancy testing. Referral for
termination of pregnancy. Smear tests.
HIV counselling and testing referred
to GUM services.

The Men's Room provides condoms,
advice and counselling.

Information/advice line with recorded
family planning services.

Work in local schools when requested.

■ Appropriateness and accessibility
Services advertised by bus
advertisements, university wall
planner, student magazine and
through work in schools. Also via
GPs and cards.

Consultations on drop-in basis.

Clinics held at three venues, two
evenings each week. General family
planning clinic every Saturday
morning. The Men's Room is open
one evening a week.

Easy access by public transport.

Confidentiality protocols, including a
form for young people to sign if they
do not wish letters to be sent home or
to their GP.

Links with schools, police, social
workers, education authority and via
health fairs and local festivals. Links
with several multi-agency forums.

■ Evaluation
Occasional surveys of users, regarding
waiting times, satisfaction and clinic
practices. Korner

■ Contact
Margaret Barnett
Family Planning Services
Administrator
Burmantofts Health Centre
Cromwell Mount
Leeds LS9 6PT

Tel: 0113 248 4330

Written or telephone enquiries.

Streetwise, Newcastle upon Tyne

■ Setting
Urban. Voluntary project with own
premises.

■ Principal aims and objectives
To empower young people by
offering both general and specialised
information, advice and support.
To enable young people to make
informed choices about their lives.
To provide a one-stop, multi-purpose
resource for young people aged 13–25
in the north-east.

■ Services offered
Staffing. 3 full-time project workers
and a full-time project coordinator.
Contraception and sexual health
sessions: 1 physician, 1 nurse,
1 receptionist/clerk and 3 project
workers to welcome and talk with
young people. Substance use session:
senior occupational therapist,
psychiatrist from drug and alcohol
services. Jobs, schemes and study
session.

Advice/counselling. Provided
throughout the week on any issue.

Contraception and sexual-health session provided by all staff present but with referral for any follow-up work.

Contraception/sexual-health services. Wide range of contraceptive services including condoms, strong condoms, lubricant and female condom. On-the-spot pregnancy testing. Referral for termination of pregnancy (staff will accompany young woman if necessary). Emergency contraception. Smear tests. Sexually transmitted disease and HIV testing referred to GUM services (staff will accompany young person).

Drop-in service. General information and advice sessions; drug, alcohol and solvent misuse session; jobs, schemes and study session. Group for pregnant young women supported by two midwives (health visitor and family planning trained).

Drug session. Prescriptions. Informal provision for the younger users, and general access throughout the week.

Work in youth clubs, youth training schemes and schools. Targeting young black people and young deaf people.

■ Appropriateness and accessibility

Services advertised by posters and leaflets. *Yellow Pages.* Press and media coverage and word of mouth.

Consultations offered on drop-in basis. Appointments for follow-up.

Dedicated premises above a shop in centre of town. Access from all areas of city by bus/metro.

Contraception and sexual health sessions offered three days a week in the early and late afternoons.

Drinks available. Music. Health promotion information.

Confidentiality a priority. Action taken only with the informed consent of the young person.

Counselling service offers a choice of male/female, lesbian/gay or black counsellors. All counselling is client-led; young people known only by first name; no time limit on how long or how often they attend; drop-in access for crisis needs.

Links and partnerships with multi-agency management committee: careers service, drugs prevention service, community health council, sexual health manager, lawyer, social services HIV prevention worker, advice worker, GUM services, health information phoneline, substance misuse team and the youth service. Joint work with young people's advisory centre.

■ Evaluation

Comments sheet in toilets. Monitor all project users and produce annual report of activities and statistics. External evaluation underway. Focus group work with young people who provide feedback of services and needs. Occasional case studies. Korner with fuller in-house details.

■ Contact

Cullagh Warnock, Iram Shah,
 Ian Robinson, Pam Douglas
Project Staff
Streetwise
35–37 Groat Market
Newcastle Upon Tyne NE1 1UQ

Tel: 0191 230 5400
Fax: 0191 221 1722

Written or telephone enquiries. Visits by arrangement only.

Adolescent Clinics and Young People's Clinic, Ripon

■ Setting
Rural. GP practice.

■ Principal aims and objectives
To promote the health of young people. To provide user-friendly open door, confidential approach to information and advice for young people on factors that affect their health (diet, smoking, drugs). To increase knowledge and minimise adverse health consequences of sexual activity. To assist young people in building their self-esteem. To immunise against diptheria, tetanus and polio. To give young people the opportunity to build an independent relationship with practice staff.

■ Services offered
Staffing. Practice nurse, health visitor and receptionist. GP available.

Advice/counselling. Provided by nurses and doctor. Referral of under 16s where appropriate to child psychotherapy. Links with community mental health team and drug project in Harrogate.

Contraception/sexual-health services. Provided on a drop-in and appointment basis by the female GP. Pregnancy tests. Referral for termination of pregnancy.

When patients are 10 years old, health session about periods and bullying, alongside rubella immunisation.

When patients are 14 years old, individually invited to take part in a series of health sessions. The first is a Health Rave, followed by two sessions each on drugs/alcohol, sexual health and building self-esteem.

When patients are 15 years old, invited by phone for their school-leaving booster, which is combined with a health check and talk.

Weekly young people's exercise class.

Work in one secondary school as part of sex education programme.

■ Appropriateness and accessibility
Services are advertised via invitation to all young people on GP list at specific ages.

Consultations offered on drop-in and appointment basis.

Drinks available at health-check sessions.

Located in centre of town.

Confidentiality discussed.

Work in schools and youth clubs by school nurse. Staff represented on HIV strategy group.

■ Evaluation
Questionnaire before and after health checks. Some informal feedback via 'feelings' sessions.

■ Contact
Liz Booth/Margaret Millar
Practice Nurse/Health Visitor
The Surgery
Park Street
Ripon
Yorkshire HG4 2BE

Tel: 01765 692366
Fax: 01765 606440

Written enquiries preferred with SAE and any photocopying costs.

Written or telephone enquiries. Visits by arrangement only.

The Grapevine, South Shields

■ Setting
Urban. Health centre.

Principal aims and objectives
To develop broad links across a range of services and meet the Health of the Nation targets for young people in relation to unplanned pregnancy and STDs. To monitor on a six-monthly basis local numbers of conceptions and attendances at GUM clinic.

■ Services offered
Staffing. 1 physician, 2 nurses, 1 health adviser, 2 youth workers, 1 receptionist/clerk.

Advice/counselling. By nurse, doctor, health adviser on sexual-health issues. Youth workers conduct more generic work, e.g. truancy, bullying, home, relationships, schools.

Contraceptive/sexual-health services. A wide range of contraceptives including condoms, strong condoms, lubricant, after-sex emergency contraception. On-the-spot pregnancy testing, referral for termination of pregnancy. Smear and chlamydia tests. STD screening with direct access to GUM services and support from health adviser at youth session.

■ Appropriateness and accessibility
Services advertised as widely as possible: pharmacies, schools, GPs, libraries, hospitals, youth justice, social services, youth projects, children's homes. Also advertised in phone book, newspaper, cinema magazine.

Clinics located in local health centre.

Open one weekday late afternoon.

Signposting in health centre. Drinks and music available, with wide variety of health promotion information. Youth workers to talk with.

Confidentiality discussed at first visit.

Close links with GUM services, family planning services, education, obstetric/gynaecology directorate, child health, community paediatrician, GPs and Streetlevel (offering support for people with HIV/AIDS and needle exchange). Involved in multi-agency forums and Sex Action Group.

■ Evaluation
Evaluation form (confidential). Korner, plus additional information.

■ Contact
Dr Janet Gallagher SCM,
Contraception and Sexual Health
  Service
Stanhope Parade Health Centre
Gordon Street
South Shields
Tyne and Wear NE34 4JP

Tel: 0191 456 8821
Fax: 0191 427 6009

Written or telephone enquiries welcome.

Family Planning Service, Queensway Health Centre, Hatfield

■ **Setting**
Urban. Health clinics.

■ **Principal aims and objectives**
To encourage young people to use existing family planning services. To publicise the availability of such services through work undertaken with young people in schools.

■ **Services offered**
Staffing. 1 physician, 2 nurses, 2 receptionists/clerks, counsellor available as required.

Advice/counselling. Provided on sexual and reproductive health. One-off and ongoing sessions. Referral for specialist pre- and post-termination of pregnancy counselling.

Contraceptive/sexual-health services. All methods available including dual method. On-the-spot pregnancy testing. After-sex emergency contraception. Smear tests.

Some work undertaken in local schools and at health fairs.

Information line (office number) giving details of all clinics in east Hertfordshire.

■ **Appropriateness and accessibility**
Service advertised via school nurses and health visitors.

Consultations offered by appointment and on drop-in basis.

Service available one evening a week and one morning a month.

■ **Evaluation**
Full family planning and Korner statistics kept. Staff audit meetings held twice yearly. Various topics audited.

■ **Contact**
Dr Brenda Bean
Senior Clinical Medical Officer
East Hertfordshire NHS Trust
Parkway Health Clinic
Birdcroft Road
Welwyn Garden City AL8 6JE

Tel: 01707 324 541
Fax: 01707 324 541
(please telephone first)

Telephone contact preferred. Clinic based in Hatfield.

City and Hackney Young People's Services, London

■ **Setting**
Urban. Health centres.

Principal aims and objectives
To ensure that all young people have the opportunity to develop their skills and knowledge, explore their attitudes, and to make informed choices about sexual health. To improve access to sexual-health services for all young people aged under 26 in Hackney

and the City of London. To provide training and support for professionals working with young people so as to enable them better to meet young people's sexual-health needs.

Services offered

Staffing. Brook: 1 physician, 1 nurse, 1 counsellor, 1 administrative/clerical worker per session; Monday, Thursday evening, Saturday morning – contraception and counselling service. *Choices*: 1 physician, 2 nurses, 1 male worker, 1 health worker, 2 receptionists; Wednesday evening – contraception, pregnancy testing, young men's worker. *Young Men's Choices*: 1 nurse, 1 health worker, 1 counsellor; Monday evening – information and support on sexual health issues, condoms and lubricant, counselling service. *Choices N4*: 2 physicians, 2 nurses, 2 health advisers, 2 receptionists; Thursday evening – contraception, testing and treatment for STDs, HIV testing, counselling in sexual health issues.

Advice/counselling. On a wide range of sexual-/reproductive-health concerns, with referral as necessary. Short-term counselling offered.

Contraception/sexual-health services. Wide range including oral contraception, condoms and dual method. On-the-spot pregnancy testing. Referral for termination of pregnancy. Smear tests. After-sex emergency contraception. STD testing and treatment offered at Choices N4.

Wide range of activities in schools, colleges and the community, including work with young men, with lesbian/gay youth project and with black/ethnic minority communities.

Appropriateness and accessibility

Services located at health centres. Available early evening and Saturday (Brook). Good public transport access.

Good disabled access.

Drinks available. Health promotion materials.

Consultations offered on drop-in basis.

Service promoted via leaflets/posters/laminated cards. Outreach to schools, colleges and youth service to enhance young people's awareness of services offered. Listed in the *Thomson Directory*.

Policy on confidentiality explained.

Close working relationships with GUM services, health promotion, local education authorities, youth services, GPs and local HIV team. Participate in Sex Education Partnership bringing together local authority, health promotion and health service workers.

Evaluation

Information collected on numbers and reasons for attendance. Suggestions boxes and occasional user satisfactions surveys. Facilitator evaluation and occasional participant observation used for education and outreach work. Korner.

Contact

Gill Heathcote
Lead Development Worker
CHYPS
Room 312, St Leonards Primary Care Centre
Nuttall Street
Hackney
London N1 5LZ

Tel: 0171 301 3453
Fax: 0171 301 3404

Written and telephone enquiries.

KISS (Keep It Safe and Sexy), London Brook Advisory Centre, London

■ Setting
Urban. Youth complex.

■ Principal aims and objectives
To prevent and mitigate the suffering caused by unwanted pregnancy by educating young persons in matters of sex and contraception, and developing among them a sense of responsibility in regard to sexual behaviour. To inform and enable clients to negotiate safer sex and to be able to ask for what they want/need.

■ Services offered
Staffing. 1 centre manager, 1 physician, 1 nurse, 2 detached youth workers, 1 counsellor.

Advice/counselling. One-off and short-term sessions on a range of sexual and relationship matters. Specialised pregnancy counselling and for under 16s.

Contraceptive/sexual-health services. A wide range of services including condoms and other methods of contraception. On-the-spot pregnancy testing, referral for termination of pregnancy. After-sex emergency contraception. Smear tests.

Work in local schools linked particularly to sex education.

Work in adjacent youth centre/coffee bar.

Information/advice line.

■ Appropriateness and accessibility
Service promoted via posters and leaflets, advertisements in newspapers, magazines distributed in discotheques, youth workers/services and word of mouth.

Consultations offered by appointment and on drop-in basis.

Dedicated young people's service. Open Saturday afternoons.

Good public transport access. Located in high street shopping area. Clear and well-publicised written statement on confidentiality.

Good links with local schools and youth services, HIV and sexual-health services, GUM services and health promotion services.

Coffee bar and pool table in adjacent well-used youth centre.

■ Evaluation
Detailed records kept concerning each consultation (age, services supplied, referral, etc.). Korner. Client questionnaire survey. Publicised complaints procedure. End of year evaluation planned for 1995.

■ Contact
Karen Bowden
Senior Centres Manager
233 Tottenham Court Road
London W1P 9AE

Tel: 0171 580 2991
Fax: 0171 580 6740

Telephone contact initially (11 a.m. – 6.30 p.m. daily). Occasional open afternoons (by appointment only). Clinic based in Uxbridge.

Well Men's Service, London

■ Setting
Urban. Health centre.

■ Principal aims and objectives
Within the context of Health of the

Nation targets, to reduce rates of unwanted teenage pregnancy, HIV and gonorrhoea. To meet the sexual health needs of young men through the provision of services for contraception and STD prevention including hepatitis B and HIV. To promote the psychosexual health of young men. To promote genital (testicular and prostate) health among young men.

■ Services offered

Staffing. 1 clinic coordinator (nurse), 1 male nurse, 1 male receptionist.

Advice/counselling. On sexuality, sexual health, general health and lifestyles, including stress reduction. Crisis counselling and ongoing counselling for two/three sessions. HIV-related counselling and testing referred to local GUM services.

Contraceptive/sexual-health services. Wide range of services including condoms, emergency contraceptive advice.

Work undertaken in local schools, colleges and universities. Joint activities with health promotion service and gay outreach worker.

Links with occupational health services of local employers.

■ Appropriateness and accessibility

Service advertised by means of leaflets and posters as well as word of mouth.

Consultation on appointment and drop-in basis. Service available Saturday mornings.

Clear and well-publicised statement of confidentiality.

Good links with local health promotion services, GUM services, GPs and local hospitals.

Comfortable seating; television and video; drinks available.

■ Evaluation

Records kept of numbers of clients using the service, age, area of residence, etc. Customer services survey completed by external consultants. Occasional service user questionnaires.

■ Contact

Justin Gaffney
Nurse Practitioner, Male Sexual
  Health
Well Men's Clinic
Pound Lane Clinic
London NW10 2HH

Tel: 0181 459 5116

Telephone contact.

Young People's Service, Harrow

■ Setting

Urban. Health centre.

■ Principal aims and objectives

To provide advice on sexual health and contraception. To provide a comprehensive range of contraception methods. To provide counselling services. To provide a rapid pregnancy testing and diagnosis service. To ensure the needs of young people, male and female, are met. To ensure that the services provided are confidential, non-judgemental, easily accessible and widely advertised.

■ Services offered

Staffing. 1 physician, 2 nurses, 2 clerical/reception staff per clinic session. 1 nurse specialist per drop-in session.

Advice/counselling. Provided on a wide range of family planning and sexual health issues. Specialist counselling by trained staff for young people experiencing emotional, psychological or behavioural problems. Ongoing counselling needs referred to psychology department at Northwick Park Hospital.

Contraceptive/sexual-health services. Wide range of contraceptive services including condoms and dual method. On-the-spot pregnancy tests. Referral for termination of pregnancy. After-sex emergency contraception. Smear tests.

Wide range of outreach activities including roadshow exhibitions in local libraries and shopping centres and health fairs. Work in local schools, youth clubs and youth centres.

■ **Appropriateness and accessibility**
Service advertised via the *Thomson Directory*, displays/roadshows in libraries, health centres, schools, youth clubs. Leaflets distributed via Community Health Council and other means.

Consultations offered by appointment and on drop-in basis.

Three dedicated young people's sessions per week, but young people welcome at all sessions. Drop-in sessions run by specialist nurse. Open three days a week after school hours and Saturday mornings. Magazines and music available in waiting area.

Services mainly located at one centre, Caryl Thomas Clinic. Plans to relocate to a dedicated centre in the centre of Harrow.

Good links with GUM services, drug and alcohol services, obstetrics and gynaecology, gay and lesbian helpline.

■ **Evaluation**
Audit records. Korner. Recent evaluation of family planning service including young people's provision. User survey. Local schools' survey concerning knowledge of clinic services.

■ **Contact**
Dr Bela Reed
Senior Clinical Medical Officer
Community Gynaecology Services
Northwick Park Hospital
Watford Road
Harrow HA1 3UJ

Tel: 0181 869 2907
Fax: 0181 732 2877

Written enquiries.

Young Person's Health Advice Service, Romford and Barking

■ **Setting**
Urban/suburban. Youth Information Shop (Romford). Health centre (Barking).

■ **Principal aims and objectives**
To work to meet local Health of the Nation targets to reduce unintended pregnancy and to contribute to STD prevention. To provide an accessible and user-friendly service.

■ **Services offered**
Staffing. 1 physician, 1 nurse, 1 counsellor, 2 receptionists, 1 outreach worker. Information workers at Information Shop.

Advice/counselling. Crisis and short-term. Can provide pre-HIV-test counselling. Referral for ongoing counselling.

Contraception/sexual-health services. Wide range including condoms (extra strong available) and after-sex emergency contraception. Smear tests. On-the-spot pregnancy testing. Referral for termination of pregnancy.

Outreach across three boroughs on streets and in schools, colleges and youth clubs. Support and information provided.

Recorded information on answering machine.

■ Appropriateness and acceptability

Advertised via information cards, newspapers, radio. Also at nightclubs and in youth centres. Publicity gained through winning Healthy Alliance Award.

Services open some weekdays late afternoon/early evening.

Good public transport access.

Confidentiality statement on all publicity.

Offers advice and support on range of health issues, not only family planning.

Good links with youth service, statutory and voluntary mental health organisations, Child and Family Health Consultation Group, GPs.

Good relationship with local press.

■ Evaluation

Monitoring of numbers of young people using service and feedback from young people. Korner.

■ Contact

Gina Burgess
Senior Health Promotion Officer
BHB Community Healthcare Centre
Health Promotion and AIDS Services
Cherry Ward, High Wood Hospital
Ongar Road
Brentwood
Essex CM 15 9DY

Tel: 01277 232450
Fax: 01277 229102

Written or telephone enquiries.
Visits by arrangement.

NORTH WEST

Wirral Brook Advisory Centre, Birkenhead

■ Setting
Medium-sized town. Dedicated advisory centre.

■ Principal aims and objectives
To maintain and improve the sexual health of young people. To provide a range of contraceptive services appropriate to young people's needs.

■ Services offered
Staffing. Minimum of 1 doctor, 1 nurse, 1 counsellor and 1 receptionist per session.

Advice/counselling. On contraceptive and sexual-health needs, pre- and post-termination of pregnancy. Referral for HIV-related counselling and testing, for STD services and for drug-related services.

Contraception/sexual-health services. Range of contraceptive services including strong condoms. On-the-spot pregnancy tests. After-sex emergency contraception. Smear tests. Referral for termination of pregnancy.

Education officer attached to centre undertakes work with local schools/youth centres.

■ Appropriateness and accessibility
Located in self-contained premises in town centre near to McDonalds.

Posters, music, drinks, box of toys for children, pram spot, disabled access and health promotion materials for young people.

Service advertised through high-profile displays in town centre (e.g. on St Valentine's Day), Condom Cavaliers activities in local discotheques and nightclubs, youth services and young people's grapevine.

Times of clinics or drop-in service available by telephone.

Service offered weekdays after school hours. Saturday clinic.

■ Evaluation
Service monitored formally and informally. Service-use statistics published in annual report. Korner. Ongoing consumer satisfaction survey. Well-advertised complaints procedure.

■ Contact
Jean Rust
Centre Manager
Wirral Brook Advisory Service
14 Whetstone Lane
Charing Cross
Birkenhead L41 2QR

Tel: 0151 670 0177
Fax: 0151 670 0209

Contact by letter or telephone (12 p.m. – 4 p.m.). Visits possible. Donations welcome; charge may be made depending on length of visit and input/information required.

Teenage Advisory Clinic, Bolton

■ Setting
Urban. Health clinic.

■ Principal aims and objectives
To reach/involve young people who are sexually active. To increase access to the service and uptake of contraception. To reduce the abortion and unplanned pregnancy rates. To undertake health promotion.

■ Services offered
Staffing. 1 doctor, 2 nurses, 2 receptionists, 1 outreach worker.

Advice/counselling. Provided by doctor or nurse on contraception, unintended pregnancy and STDs.

Contraception/sexual-health services. Include oral contraception, condoms (including extra strong), cap and diaphragm, after-sex emergency contraception. On-the-spot pregnancy tests. Referral for termination of pregnancy.

Telephone line providing information and advice on emergency contraception.

Testing for chlamydia, referral to GUM services for other STDs and HIV.

Outreach service based in housing estate community centre. Services provided at Homeless Centre include oral contraception and condoms, emergency contraception, pregnancy testing, information and advice.

■ Appropriateness and accessibility
Service advertised on buses, in schools (stickers and brochures), to students (advert in student diary) and in youth clubs.

Service based in town centre health service facilities. Teenage Advisory Health Clinic acts as a drop-in service, open Friday late afternoon/early evening and Saturday afternoon. Music. Young people can be seen in twos or threes. Very good public transport.

Telephone information/advice line open 24 hours a day, seven days a week.

Clear statement of confidentiality.

Well-developed links with schools, social workers and youth workers.

Outreach service contacts homeless mothers, families and young men.

■ Evaluation
Evaluation forms completed by teachers and pupils in schools. Monitoring of client use. Korner.

■ Contact
Judi Noden
Senior Nurse, Family Planning
Women's Health Care
Bolton General Hospital
Minerva Road
Farnworth
Bolton BL4 0JR

Tel: 01204 390390
Fax: 01204 390525
(mark fao Judi Noden)

Telephone enquiries preferred. Visits by prior arrangement.

Tameside Young People's Health Clinic and Peer Education Project, Denton
Also known as Duke Street Clinic/Young People's Clinic

■ Setting
Urban/suburban. Youth centre.

■ Principal aims and objectives
To provide a comprehensive sexual-health service to young people.
To assist in the development of sexual-health services and peer sex education to young people.

■ Services offered
Staffing. 1 doctor, 2 nurses, 1 health adviser, 2 youth workers/full- and part-time Peer Education Project workers, 2 receptionists (both are young people from Peer Education Project). 1 full-time and 1 part-time Peer Education Project worker.

Advice/counselling. Provided by trained youth workers. HIV pre-test counselling available. Outreach work undertaken in schools and youth centres to improve links with the clinic. An answering machine provides telephone information.

Contraception/sexual-health services. Include oral contraception, condoms (including extra strong), female condoms, cap/diaphragm, after-sex emergency contraception. On-the-spot pregnancy testing. Smear tests. Referral for termination of pregnancy.

■ Appropriateness and accessibility
Service advertised via leaflets and posters. Clinic open Monday late afternoon/early evening. Pregnancy tests available throughout the week. Peer Education Project runs each day.

Drop-in and telephone appointments. Clinic located within established youth centre on main bus route.

Young people's access clinic for those aged 11–25 (main priority 13–16-year-olds).

Strict policy on confidentiality advertised on all publicity material.

Peer Education Project works in schools, colleges and youth clubs. Peer educators specialise in work in areas such as contraception, peer pressure, rape, pregnancy, relationships, HIV and drugs.

Links with schools and strategy forums (young people, HIV/AIDS and sex education).

■ Evaluation
Consultation with users and staff. Suggestions box. Korner.

■ Contact
Tim Smith/Glynnis Francis
Clinic Coordinator/Youth Worker
Duke Street Young People's Centre
Duke Street
Denton M34 2AN

Tel: 0161 320 8918 (clinic)
      0161 336 6615 (office)
Fax: 0161 367 8229

Written or telephone enquiries. Visits by prior arrangement.

Merseyside Brook Advisory Centre, Liverpool

■ Setting
Inner city area. Dedicated advisory centre.

■ Principal aims and objectives
Prevention and mitigation of the suffering caused by unwanted pregnancy by educating young persons in matters of sex and contraception and developing among them a sense of responsibility with regard to sexual behaviour.

Services offered

Staffing. 1 doctor, 2–3 nurses, 1 counsellor, 2 receptionists (main sessions); 2 nurses, 2 receptionists (nurse administered sessions).

Advice/counselling. To all new clients. Pregnancy counselling. Referral for termination of pregnancy. Referral to GUM services for STD advice and testing plus HIV-related support. Advice on health education issues.

Contraception/sexual-health services. Range of contraceptive services including condoms (including extra-strong) and dual methods. After-sex emergency contraception. Smear tests.

Group work undertaken in local schools and youth clubs to enhance awareness of service among teachers, youth workers and potential service users.

Appropriateness and accessibility

Centrally located in busy shopping area.

Pram spot, disabled access.

Promoted through posters in colleges and universities, through advertising cards giving name and telephone number, and through grapevine.

Sessions held at a wide variety of times, but including after-school hours and Saturday morning. Drop-in service.

Clearly stated policy on confidentiality

Evaluation

Regular monitoring of service users and patterns of service use. Korner. Audits of specific aspects of service provision.

Contact

Sue Ryrie or Liz Hall
Manager/Education Officer
Merseyside Brook Advisory Centre
104 Bold Street
Liverpool L1 4HY

Tel: 0151 709 4558 (Mon, Tues, Thurs, Fri)
Fax: 0151 709 4558 (ring first)

Letter and telephone enquiries welcome. Visits can be arranged with prior notice.

Young People's Family Planning Clinic, Macclesfield

Setting

Small town with rural feeder areas. Health clinic.

Principal aims and objectives

To provide an accessible service to young people on all aspects of sexual health. To promote individual control over fertility. To minimise the adverse effects of sexual activity. To support those in need of help and advice for sexual- and reproductive-health problems. To promote the rewarding expression of sexuality and satisfying emotional relationships.

Services offered

Staffing. 1 doctor, 1 nurse, 1 youth worker and 1 receptionist at each session.

Advice/counselling. Basic counselling/advice provided by youth worker with referral if necessary. Pre- and post-termination of pregnancy counselling.

Contraception/sexual-health services. Condoms and other contraceptive services. On-the-spot pregnancy testing. After-sex emergency contraception. Smear tests. STD tests via laboratory services. Referral for termination of pregnancy.

Some work undertaken with schools and youth clubs.

■ Appropriateness and accessibility

Service promoted by local school nurses and personal and social education coordinators. Leaflets advertising service available in libraries, colleges, leisure centre, youth centres/services.

Consultation on drop-in and appointment basis. Service offered one day a week in after-school hours.

Policy on confidentiality explained on first visit.

Out-of-hours, recorded message service giving doctor's home telephone number for emergency service.

■ Evaluation

Service monitored through responses on patient data collection forms. Small survey of service users conducted. Korner. Other approaches to evaluation being considered.

■ Contact

Dr Lesley Batchelor
Senior Clinical Medical Officer
Macclesfield District Hospital
Family Planning
Victoria Road
Macclesfield SK10 3BL

Tel: 01625 661169
Fax: 01625 663305

The Youth Advice Shop, Warrington

■ Setting

Youth advice shop/services in urban area.

■ Principal aims and objectives

To reduce unwanted teenage pregnancies and control the spread of HIV. To offer help, advice and counselling in relation to sexual behaviour. To provide positive health messages concerning safer sexual practices. To give advice and contraceptive supplies as appropriate.

■ Services offered

Staffing. 1 doctor, 1 nurse and a minimum of 2 youth workers per session.

Advice/basic counselling. On a one-off basis offered by youth workers. Referral to specialist agencies as appropriate.

Contraception/sexual-health services. Condoms and other contraceptive services. On-the-spot pregnancy tests. After-sex emergency contraception. Referral for termination of pregnancy.

Travelling Youth Advice Shop Service visits colleges and youth centres, as requested, to provide information and advice on family planning and sexual health.

■ Appropriateness and accessibility

Located in self-contained accommodation above shops in town centre.

Centrally located close to public transport.

Service promoted through youth service and Travelling Youth Advice Shop, school nurses and GPs, colleges and universities, and via the phone book.

Drop-in service late afternoon/evening four nights a week plus Saturday afternoons.

Clear and well-publicised policy on confidentiality.

Links with local AIDS line, Lifeline (drugs), homelessness group, community drugs project and Rape Crisis service.

Healthy Alliance between Warrington Community Health Care NHS Trust, Cheshire Youth Service and North Cheshire Health.

■ Evaluation

Information collected on service provided. Korner. Written evaluation report.

■ Contact

Trish Reid
Service Coordinator
Youth Advice Shop
37–39 Buttermarket Street
Warrington WA1 2LY

Tel: 01925 231880

Written enquiries preferred.

SOUTH AND WEST

The Junction Health Advisory Centre, Bournemouth

■ **Setting**
Urban. Youth advisory centre.

■ **Principal aims and objectives**
To improve the sexual health of young people through health promotion activity. To provide young people with the skills to access general health care. To reduce rates of unwanted pregnancy among young people in relation to Health of the Nation targets.

■ **Services offered**
Staffing. 1 doctor, 1 nurse, 1 in-house counsellor, 1 receptionist.

Assessment/counselling. Provided by nurse with referral to specialist counselling/advice services as necessary.

Contraception/sexual-health services. Condoms (including strong) and other contraceptive services. On-the-spot pregnancy tests. After-sex emergency contraception. Referral for termination of pregnancy.

Work undertaken with local schools and youth clubs.

■ **Appropriateness and accessibility**
Located in established multi-agency youth centre offering advice, counselling and support to young people.

Close to public transport.

Appointment and drop-in service in out-of-school hours and on Saturday morning.

Clear and well-publicised statement of confidentiality

Work supported by a youth advisory forum meeting every six/eight weeks.

Joint advertising with other youth advisory services.

■ **Evaluation**
Some monitoring of service use. Korner.

■ **Contact**
Pat Palmer, Family Planning
  Nurse/Health Adviser
The Junction
266 Holdenhurst Road
Bournemouth BH8 8AY

Tel: 01202 683363
Fax: 01202 667009

Written enquiries preferred.

Young Adults' Drop-in Clinic, Burnham-on-Sea

■ **Setting**
Small town. GP health centre.

■ **Principal aims and objectives**
Through ongoing support and education to provide young people with an opportunity to take responsibility for their own behaviour,

health care and lifestyle. To facilitate self-reliance, self-discipline and responsibility among young adults by providing a service where all health issues can be discussed in complete confidence.

■ Services offered
Staffing. 1 doctor, 1 nurse, 1 receptionist.

Advice/counselling. On a range of health problems including contraception, safer sex, eating disorders, substance use. Referral to specialist agencies as appropriate.

Contraception/sexual-health services. Condoms (including extra strong) and other contraceptive services. On the spot pregnancy tests. After-sex emergency contraception. Smear tests. Referral for termination of pregnancy. Referral for STDs including HIV antibody testing.

■ Appropriateness and accessibility
Drop-in service one evening per week.

Publicity via local youth services and churches as well as GPs in the local area/region, posters, leaflets and word of mouth.

■ Evaluation
Mini-audit recently completed. Suggestions box. Survey in local schools planned.

■ Contact
Heather Litton
Senior Practice Nurse
Burnham Medical Centre
Love Lane
Burnham-on-Sea TA8 1EU

Tel: 01278 795445
Fax: 01278 793024

Written enquiries preferred initially. Visits by appointment only.

Healthwise, Coleford Health Centre, Gloucester
(Health advice for the under 25s)

■ Setting
Rural. Health centre.

■ Principal aims and objectives
Comprehensive service to provide advice, information and resources to promote young people's physical, emotional and sexual health. Emphasis on skills training for young people and health professionals. Service established following local needs assessment and in relation to the attainment of Health of the Nation targets.

■ Services offered
Staffing. 2 physicians, 2 nurses, 1 youth worker, 1 receptionist.

Advice/counselling. Provided by centre-based youth worker. Referrals for HIV-related testing and support, and for other specialised needs.

Contraception/sexual-health services. Include condoms (including extra strong), IUDs. On-the-spot pregnancy tests, after-sex emergency contra-ception, smear tests. Referrals for termination of pregnancy.

Work in local schools and colleges. Includes work with young people with learning difficulties and physically disabled young people.

■ Appropriateness and accessibility
Service advertised through local newspapers (including free news-papers), Radio Gloucestershire, parish magazine and local health promotion telephone line.

Consultations offered both on drop-in basis and by appointment.

Dedicated young people's service open out-of-school hours (Friday 4 p.m.–6 p.m.). Music, youth magazines and drinks available in reception area. Disabled access.

Clear statement of confidentiality.

Well-developed links with local GPs, relevant hospital services, schools and youth services.

■ Evaluation
Range of techniques used, including records of number and type of clinic attenders, 'pen pictures' of service users, daybook with general comments. Korner.

■ Contact
Dr Pauline Allen
Manager and Head of Family
  Planning Services
Hope House
Gloucestershire Royal Hospital
Gloucester GL1 3NN

Tel: 01452 395999
Fax: 01452 394808

Written enquiry preferred.

Community Clinics for Young People, Southampton, Shirley New Milton, Romsey and Thornhill

■ Setting
Urban area. Health centre/youth club/community hall/leisure complex.

■ Principal aims and objectives
To reduce the rate of unwanted teenage pregnancies and the incidence of STDs through the provision of a full range of contraceptive and other sexual health services. To provide advice/counselling on sexual health. To encourage safer sexual practice and the use of dual methods. To address general health issues including drugs, diet and smoking.

■ Services offered
Staffing. 1 physician, 1 nurse, 1 receptionist/clerk, 1 youth worker per session.

Advice/counselling. Provided on a range of sexual and reproductive health topics at one main centre (Hamtun Youth and Advisory Service, Shirley) and three satellite centres (New Milton, Romsey, Thornhill). Pre- and post-termination of pregnancy counselling. Counselling/advice on the management of PMT. Referral for psychosexual counselling.

Contraceptives/sexual-health services. Wide range of services including dual method. On-the-spot pregnancy testing. Referral for termination of pregnancy. After-sex emergency contraception. Smear tests. Referral for HIV testing.

Work undertaken in local schools and youth clubs. Street-based youth work. Work undertaken at health fairs and summer community concerts.

Information/advice line offered five days a week.

■ Appropriateness and accessibility
Service advertised through posters, advertising cards, health fairs, telephone book and local newspaper. Outreach workers and health promotion services publicise the existence of the young people's clinics.

Consultations by appointment and on drop-in basis.

Services available early evening four days a week at main centre and one day a week at satellites.

Music, videos, coffee/tea in reception area. Games and discussions while young people are waiting in clinic.

Clear and well-publicised statement of confidentiality.

Links with health promotion/sexual health workers. Links with local GUM services and drugs advisory service.

Participation in range of local young people's forums.

■ Evaluation
Client satisfaction survey. Feedback from sessions conducted in schools. Korner. Major evaluation planned for January 1996.

■ Contact
Rosalie Gurr or Alison Milchem
Family Planning Services
  Manager/Youth Outreach Nurse
Family Planning Services
Central Health Clinic
East Park Terrace
Southampton SO14 0YL

Tel: 01703 634321
Fax: 01703 634375

Written enquiries in the first instance.

Sex Sense, Portsmouth

■ Setting
Urban/suburban. Health centres/youth centres.

■ Principal aims and objectives
To provide young people with information, advice and support beneficial to sexual health. To provide sex education in schools, colleges, universities and youth clubs. To assist in the attainment of Health of the Nation targets.

■ Services offered
Staffing. 6 doctors, 6 nurses, 3 full-time project workers.

Advice/counselling. Single-session counselling on variety of topics, with referral as necessary.

Contraception/sexual-health services. Condoms (including extra-strong condoms) and other contraceptives. After-sex emergency contraception. Referral for termination of pregnancy and for GUM problems.

Outreach work with young people, including young homeless people, sex workers and ethnic minority youth groups.

Wide range of posters, leaflets and other publicity/promotional materials developed.

Sex education in schools, colleges and youth clubs.

Health promotion activities in shopping centres, nightclubs and family centres.

■ Appropriateness and accessibility
Service name suggested by young people.

Service offered in a range of neutral settings including clinics, youth clubs and voluntary youth projects.

Access well signposted; refreshments provided; disabled access in most settings.

Clear and publicised policy on confidentiality.

Project workers actively publicise service and encourage young people to attend. About one-third of service users are male.

Strong emphasis on outreach and other activities to bring service to attention of potential users.

Service offered after school hours on weekdays.

■ Evaluation
Service monitored by the completion of standard service user form. Additional information collected by means of questionnaires distributed to young people using the service. Independent evaluation to be commissioned.

■ Contact
Sandy Prior
Manager, Sex Sense
Portsmouth Health Care NHS Trust
Family Planning and Women's Health
  Services
Ella Gordon Unit, East Wing
St Mary's Hospital
Portsmouth PO3 6AF

Tel: 01705 866503
Fax: 01705 866311

Written or telephone enquiries. Visits welcome by prior arrangement.

Cornwall Brook Advisory Centre, Redruth

■ Setting
Town in rural area. Dedicated advisory centre.

■ Principal aims and objectives
To prevent and mitigate the suffering caused by unwanted pregnancy by educating young persons in matters of sex and contraception, and developing among them a sense of responsibility with regard to sexual behaviour.

■ Services offered
Staffing. 1 physician, 1 nurse, 1 receptionist, 1 counsellor.

Advice/counselling. Offered on a wide range of sexual and reproductive concerns by counsellor at first visit and then on request. Pregnancy-test support. Pre- and post-termination of pregnancy counselling. Counselling on sexual health/relationships with referral as necessary.

Contraception/sexual-health services. Wide range of services including condoms and dual method. On-the-spot pregnancy testing. Referral for termination of pregnancy. After-sex emergency contraception. Smear tests.

Work undertaken with Young Farmers' groups, young women's groups and with young people with learning difficulties.

Group-work sessions involving young people.

Information/advice line with answering service for after-sex emergency contraception and other urgent needs.

■ Appropriateness and accessibility
Service advertised through local radio and newspapers, by health promotion officers, and through word of mouth.

Consultations offered on drop-in basis and by appointment.

Service currently offered one afternoon and one early evening per week, plus Saturday afternoons.

On bus route to leisure centre, next to large market. Direct access to dedicated premises.

Space totally devoted to young people. Health promotion posters/leaflets/information readily available.

Statement of confidentiality.

Strong links with local health promotion services, GUM services, youth workers and some GPs.

■ **Evaluation**
Comments book. Complaints procedure. Korner.

■ **Contact**
Ruth Milner-Scott
Centre Manager
Cornwall Brook Advisory Centre
60 Station Road
Pool
Redruth TR15 3QG

Tel: 01209 710088

Written or telephone enquiries. Visits welcome (advance appointment necessary).

Advisory Centre for Young People, Salisbury

■ **Setting**
Town/rural area. Health clinic.

■ **Principal aims and objectives**
To offer a free and confidential advice service to young people. To provide advice on birth control, help with unplanned pregnancies, and sexual, personal and emotional problems. To reduce the incidence of HIV infection, other STDs and unwanted pregnancies in line with Health of the Nation targets.

■ **Services offered**
Staffing. 1 doctor, 1 nurse, 1 receptionist per session, plus health adviser and specialist in GUM at weekly combined clinic.

Advice/counselling. One-off and basic counselling with referral to appropriate specialist agencies. Support before and after termination of pregnancy. HIV-related support.

Contraception/sexual-health services. Provide condoms (including extra-strong) and other contraceptive services. HIV antibody tests. On-the-spot pregnancy tests. After-sex emergency contraception. Referral for termination of pregnancy.

■ **Appropriateness and accessibility**
Located in multi-function health centre in town centre close to public transport.

After-school service two days per week with additional lunchtime combined family planning/GUM clinic.

Well established links with local health promotion services, youth and community services and Benefits Agency.

■ **Evaluation**
Initial survey of service users. Occasional questionnaires to service users. Korner.

■ **Contact**
Jan Sanders
Manager, Family Planning Services
Salisbury District Hospital
Salisbury SP2 8BJ

Tel: 01722 336262 ext. 2179
Fax: 01722 410769

Written enquiries initially.

SOUTH THAMES

Youth Advisory Clinics, Bexleyheath, Blackfen and Erith

■ Setting
Suburban. Neighbourhood health centres.

Principal aims and objectives
To meet Health of the Nation targets to reduce teenage pregnancy and STDs. To give information on sexual health – particularly HIV/AIDS. To address other issues in young people's lives. To help young people gain a sense of their own importance and of control over their lives. To specifically target young people, treat them with respect and be non-judgemental.

■ Services offered
Staffing. 1 physician, 2 nurses (1 school nurse), 2 receptionists/clerks.

Advice/counselling. By nurse with referral as necessary. Pre- and post-termination of pregnancy support.

Contraception/sexual-health services. Wide range of contraceptives including condoms, strong condoms, lubricant and after-sex emergency contraception. On-the-spot pregnancy testing. Referral for termination of pregnancy. Smear tests. HIV and other STD tests referred to GUM services.

Phoneline available throughout week via family planning clinics. Helpline at evenings and weekends offers emergency contraception information.

■ Appropriateness and accessibility
Services advertised by posters in schools, libraries, colleges and via health education unit.

Service listed in telephone book and advertised in local free newspaper.

Clinics located in neighbourhood health centres.

Drop-in sessions three evenings each week.

Music and information cassettes with headphones available in clinics.

Health promotion displays.

Confidentiality discussed at first visit.

Close links with HIV nurse from HIV unit. Member of district youth advisory group and other forums.

■ Evaluation
Consumer research when service first set up. Continue to ask young people how they heard of the clinic, what they like/do not like. Health promotion officer carries out evaluation. Korner plus greater detail.

■ Contact
Mrs Maureen Willis
Locality Nurse Manager
Pinewood House
Bexley Hospital
Bexleyheath DA5 2BW

Tel: 01322 526282 ext. 2416
Fax: 01332 556531

Written or telephone enquiries welcome.

Young People's Drop-in Clinic, Brighton

■ Setting
Urban. Health centre.

■ Principal aims and objectives
To reduce the incidence of unplanned teenage pregnancies. To provide education aimed at encouraging the use of condoms and safer sexual practices. To conduct work with young men.

■ Services offered
Staffing. 1 physician, 1 nurse, 1 counsellor, 1 receptionist/clerk plus a young voluntary worker to greet clients, 1 male youth worker.

Advice/counselling. Broad-based counselling by counsellor. Sexual health counselling/advice by nurse and doctor. Male youth worker does one-to-one sessions with young men attending. Group work – particularly male worker with young men outside of clinic times.

Contraception/sexual-health services. Including range of condoms and dual method. On-the-spot pregnancy testing. Referral for termination of pregnancy.

Youthline at YMCA provides condoms and advertises the clinic.

Outreach by clinic nurse (also school nurse), who runs a weekly session for sixth-formers. Youth worker does sexuality/sexual health work in range of settings.

■ Appropriateness and accessibility
Service widely advertised – nightclub magazine, *Yellow Pages, Talking Pages.* Wide distribution of leaflets/posters to GPs, schools, libraries, youth clubs, festival magazine and local council calendar. Leaflets/information cards for different client groups and different needs, e.g. emergency contraception, young men.

Drop-in and telephone appointments.

Clinic located in city-centre-based health centre, with good public transport access.

Clinic holds one late afternoon session, and there is a satellite clinic in rural health centre. Joint family planning session at GUM clinic one day a week – not specific to young people.

Specific protocol on confidentiality. This is advertised and discussed with each young person on first visit.

Joint work developed locally including with young women's support group, social services, youth services and voluntary youth agencies. Young people's sexual health forum established.

■ Evaluation
End of year report. Service user surveys, including one on confidentiality, and other small audits. External evaluation of one satellite clinic. Suggestions box. Korner.

■ Contact
Sue Ward
Service Manager (FPS),
Clinical Nurse
Specialist Family Planning Clinic
Morley Street Health Centre
Brighton BN2 2RA

Tel: 01273 696011 ext. 3839

Written or telephone enquiries.

Young Person's Clinic, Chatham

■ Setting
Town. Community health clinics.

Principal aims and objectives
To promote contraceptive services. To link with other services available for young people. To meet the Health of the Nation targets. To promote links between school nurses and the family planning service in order to provide a holistic service.

■ Services offered
Staffing. 1 physician, 1 nurse, 1 counsellor, 1–2 receptionists.

Advice/counselling. From medical/nursing staff on pre- and post-termination of pregnancy and on psychosexual matters. Specialist counsellor for under 20s available.

Contraception/sexual-health services. Wide range available, including dual method, and strong and female condoms. On-the-spot pregnancy testing. Smear tests. Referral for termination of pregnancy.

Referral to GUM services for STD testing. For HIV testing, referral to local HIV unit.

Outreach work on an ad-hoc basis by school nurses in schools, youth clubs, deaf society and women's refuge.

■ Appropriateness and accessibility
Services advertised via posters in schools, health centres, Youth Information Shop. Liaison via a young person's forum.

Centrally located, close to public transport and local schools.

Consultations on drop-in and appointment basis, one late afternoon each week.

Drinks available and music played during session.

Confidentiality discussed at first visit and advertised on publicity.

■ Evaluation
Qualitative surveys of young people's attitudes. Staff discuss the clinic's appropriateness with young people. Korner, including more specific data for under 16s.

■ Contact
Pauline Ruddy, Clinic Manager
Elmhouse Clinic
15 New Road Avenue
Chatham
Kent ME4 6BA

Tel: 01634 400123

Telephone or written enquiries.

Sussed Sex in 'Number 18', Chichester

■ Setting
Urban. Youth centre.

Principal aims and objectives
To provide a contact point for young people (who would not access a family planning clinic) for the supply of information, advice and contraceptive care, as well as advice on other issues – drugs, finance, etc. To make contact with younger service users. To offer an informal environment. To reduce the incidence of unplanned pregnancies.

■ Services offered
Staffing. Either 1 physician or 1 nurse. Lack of space precludes two staff members. No examination facilities – refer to nearby family planning clinic for other than the contraceptive pill,

condoms, emergency contraception. 2 youth workers.

Advice/counselling. Sexual health, condom use, safer sex – main focus is health promotion. Group work.

Work in schools.

■ Appropriateness and accessibility

Located in specialist under-18s youth centre with 1950s style coffee bar in town centre.

Good public transport.

Posters, small information cards and beer mats distributed in schools, clubs and pubs by the health promotion officer.

Drop-in service one late afternoon.

Confidentiality stressed to all young people.

Links to schools via school nurses. Multi-agency steering group, including GUM services and education department.

■ Evaluation

Korner plus further details, e.g. where users heard of the service, age of users. Informal feedback via youth worker.

■ Contact

Dr Sylvia Ellis
Senior Clinical Medical Officer,
Family Planning
Chapel Street Clinic
Chapel Street
Chichester PO19 1BX

Tel: 01243 783325

Chris Walters, Centre Manager
'No. 18', 18 Waterloo Square
Bognor Regis

Tel: 01243 865533

Written enquiries preferred.

Family Planning Services for Young People, Optimum Health Services, London

■ Setting
Urban. Health centres and dedicated premises.

■ Principal aims and objectives
Prevention and mitigation of the suffering caused by unwanted pregnancy by educating young persons in matters of sex and contraception and developing among them a sense of responsibility in regard to sexual behaviour. To provide a specific and appropriate service for young people under 20.

■ Services offered
Staffing. Minimum of 1 physician, 1 nurse, 1 receptionist per session. Brook-based service: 1 physician, 1 nurse, 1 counsellor, 1 administrative/clerical person per session. Male nurse working across the service in youth work capacity.

Advice/counselling. Basic advice on sexual matters provided in family planning clinics, with referral to Brook for specialist advice/counselling. Psychosexual counselling available in men's clinic.

Contraception/sexual-health services. Wide range of services including oral contraceptives, condoms (strong), female condom, dual method. On-the-spot pregnancy testing. Referral for termination of pregnancy and related counselling. After-sex emergency contraception (available every evening, at weekends and bank holidays). Smear tests. Domiciliary service available to young people. Referral to GUM services for HIV-related counselling and testing, and other STDs.

24-hour information line providing information on family planning service, emergency contraception, etc.

Sex education supported/undertaken in local schools.

■ Appropriateness and accessibility

Services located in a range of south London health centres and dedicated premises.

Consultations available on appointment and drop-in basis. Young people's clinics open early evening and Saturday mornings. Music/videos in waiting areas.

Well-established interpreting services for Spanish, Vietnamese and Turkish users.

Service promoted via leaflet/posters to GPs and youth-related services. Occasional advertisements in local newspapers. One-off bus advertisement. Telephone directory.

Clear statement of confidentiality.

Links with youth centres and education department. Links with local sexual-health advisory groups.

■ Evaluation

Occasional service audits. Evaluation forms for work in school. Complaints/comments box. Occasional community-based surveys. Korner.

■ Contact

Zoe Plant
Family Planning and Reproductive
   Health Nurse Manager
Optimum Health Services
Department of Family Planning and
   Reproductive Health Care
St Giles Road
London SE5 7RN

Tel: 0171 771 3330
Fax: 0171 635 1113

Written or telephone enquiries.

Under 20s Clinic and Free Condom Clinics, Derby

■ Setting
City centre and outlying towns. Health centres.

■ Principal aims and objectives
To provide a good contraceptive and counselling service (in a friendly setting) for young people to come and discuss matters that concern them – not just sexual health.

■ Services offered
Staffing. Under 20s Clinic: 1 physician, 2 nurses, 1 receptionist/ clerk, 1 youth worker at one outlying session; *Free Condom Clinic:* 2 nurses and 1 receptionist.

Advice/counselling. Offered in all centres by nurses/doctors.

Contraception/sexual-health services. At Under 20s sessions, wide range of contraceptive services including condoms and strong condoms. On-the-spot pregnancy testing and referral for termination of pregnancy. Smear tests. Some STD testing. Other STDs referred to GUM services. Free Condom Clinic provides condoms, counselling and on-the-spot pregnancy testing.

Outreach work in university, schools and night clubs. Health promotion activities such as those on World AIDS Day.

Phoneline available to family planning services office, with recorded message for information on emergency contraception out of office hours.

■ Appropriateness and accessibility
Services advertised in the telephone directory and local newspaper, and via distribution of leaflets, business cards and posters.

Consultations at Under 20s Clinic offered on drop-in basis with follow-up appointments. Drop-in consultations only at Free Condom Clinics.

Under 20s town sessions open one late afternoon per week. Outlying sessions offered one afternoon and one evening every fortnight. Free Condom Clinics open two evenings a week.

Clear code of confidentiality. First names only used in clinic.

Music. Drinks machine available.

Links to youth services, health promotion service and school nurses.

■ Evaluation
Collect own information on service use. Two consumer surveys.

■ Contact
Gloria Percival, Support Services Manager
Family Planning and Related Services
123/5 Osmaston Road
Derby DE1 2GA

Tel: 01332 363 371 ext. 281

Written enquiries preferred.

Choices, Youth Clinic and Always, Doncaster

■ Setting
Urban. Health centre and youth centre(s).

■ Principal aims and objectives
To provide young people under 18 years with a confidential sexual-health service. To provide clinical support and back-up for sexual-health education. To provide family planning and other services and appropriate counselling support. To provide a service without discrimination which values and respects the clients' own beliefs allowing them the opportunity for choice in a welcoming, comfortable and confidential environment.

■ Services offered
Staffing. Choices: 1 physician, 3 nurses, 2 receptionists/clerks, 1 youth worker; *Youth Clinic*: 1 physician, 1 nurse, 1 receptionist/clerk, 1 outreach worker; *Always*: 1 physician, 2 nurses, 1 receptionist/clerk, 1 community development worker, 1 outreach worker.

Advice/counselling. Choices: by nurse (including advice on termination of pregnancy) and youth worker (male); Youth Clinic: by youth worker; Always: by both nurses and youth worker.

Contraception/sexual-health services. Choices: wide range of services including strong condoms, female condoms, dual-method contraception. On-the-spot pregnancy testing. Referral for termination of pregnancy. After-sex emergency contraception. Smear tests. Other testing referred to GUM services. *Youth Clinic:* wide range of services available. *Always:* same as Choices, but in addition provides a wide range of information and advice on many issues which affect the health and well-being of young people. Examples include drug and alcohol abuse, bereavement counselling, benefits advice and advice on eating disorders.

Outreach by clinic staff, particularly youth and outreach workers. Work with local leaving-care scheme for young people. Links to schools, youth clubs, alcohol misuse team, drugs workers, college for the deaf, probation, street agencies, lesbian and gay organisations, homelessness workers, occupational health professionals, religious organisations and careers service. Participate in range of multi-agency forums.

Phoneline for information on emergency contraception.

■ Appropriateness and accessibility
Distributed posters, leaflets, cards/fliers via school nurses, GPs, nightclubs, colleges and post offices. Radio advertisements. Name 'Choices' chosen in a nightclub competition.

Consultations mainly on drop-in basis. Counselling by appointment.

Choices open one evening and Saturday afternoon. Youth Clinic and Always two afternoon sessions each per week. Television in waiting areas.

Policy on confidentiality clearly stated and supported by a statement on behalf of all staff on young people's rights.

■ Evaluation
Two in-house surveys. Local purchasers have conducted a survey of 1500 young people on their opinions of the health service, including sexual-health services.

Staff audit meetings every six weeks to review activities.

Touch screen satisfaction survey pilot in Choices.

'Your opinion counts' suggestions boxes in clinics.

Computerised Korner plus more in-depth information: waiting times, numbers of young people seeing youth worker, smoking, etc.

■ Contact
Janet Cozens
Family Planning Manager
Chequer Road Clinic
Doncaster
South Yorkshire DN1 2AD

Tel: 01302 367051
Fax: 01302 340587

Written or telephone enquiries. Visits by arrangement.

SHOP (Sexual Health Options Project), Ilkeston

■ Setting
Suburban town. Health centre.

■ Principal aims and objectives
To access young people, be easily available to them, and to offer advice and counselling as required in a non-threatening and non-judgemental way.

■ Services offered
Staffing. 1 physician, 2 nurses (one school nurse), 1 receptionist/clerk, 1 youth worker.

Advice/counselling. Offered by nurse, doctor and the youth worker, who will also provide ongoing support/counselling.

Contraceptive/sexual-health services. A wide range of contraceptives including condoms, strong condoms, lubricant, female condoms, after-sex emergency contraception. On-the-spot pregnancy testing, referral for termination of pregnancy direct to hospital services. Smear and chlamydia tests; HIV and other STD screening referred to GUM services.

Work in schools, further education colleges, youth clubs, discussion groups and as part of sex education programme. Outreach work in schools, further education colleges and youth clubs.

■ Appropriateness and accessibility
Services advertised by clinic youth worker and with cards.

Local newspaper. Telephone directory.

Clinic located in local health centre in centre of town.

Drop-in sessions every second and fourth Monday, late afternoon.

Music and drinks available.

Youth worker in waiting area to welcome young people.

Confidentiality discussed at first visit.

Links with youth service, school nurses, child health officers and school medical officers.

■ Evaluation
Occasional questionnaires from users. Korner.

■ Contact
Dr Jackie Abrahams
Senior Clinical Medical Officer, Family Planning
7 Penny Long Lane
Derby DE22 1AX

Tel: 01332 557696

Written or telephone enquiries welcome.

Young People's Clinic, Leicester

■ Setting
Urban. Health centre and community centre.

■ Principal aims and objectives
To work with young people to enhance their quality of life. To provide contraceptive care in a confidential and non-judgemental environment.

■ Services offered
Staffing. Health centre: 1–2 physicians (both GUM trained), 2–3 nurses (1 nurse specialist in HIV advice in midwifery), 1 nursing assistant, 2 receptionists/clerks per session. Community centre: 1 nurse and 1 nursing assistant.

Advice/counselling. Provided by doctors and nurses who are specifically chosen for their counselling skills. Doctor undertakes some pre- and post-termination of pregnancy counselling. Psychosexual counselling available through family planning services.

Contraception/sexual-health services. Wide range of contraceptive services including condoms, strong condoms, lubricant, female condoms. On-the-spot pregnancy testing. Referral for termination of pregnancy. Smear tests. Refer most STDs to GUM services but will perform STD test if young person not willing to attend GUM clinic. At community centre, sexual-health advice, condoms and pregnancy tests available.

Work in schools and youth clubs. Close links to health promotion services, where a peer education programme is based. Work with young men at risk.

Sexual-health helpline available during opening hours, plus out-of-hours recorded message service.

■ Appropriateness and accessibility
Services advertised in telephone directory. Distribution of leaflets, posters and cards via health promotion service, school nurses, community health staff and hospitals. Insert in nightclub magazine.

Consultations offered on drop-in basis.

Sessions offered one late afternoon and one mid-afternoon at city centre clinic. At local health centre, one late afternoon. At community centre, one late afternoon session. Young people supported and encouraged to use any of the family planning services.

Clear code of confidentiality with detailed staff guidelines. Training for reception staff. Confidentiality discussed with all young people at first visit and clearly advertised on all publicity.

Easy access to all clinics. Displays about specific sexual health issues.

Links to GUM services, health promotion service, school nurses and HIV coordinator. Working with purchasers developing sexual-health strategy. Forums with voluntary groups and other services.

■ Evaluation
User satisfaction survey. Korner with additional information for user profile.

■ Contact
Dr Gill Wandless
Lead Clinician, Family Planning
  Services
Family Planning Clinic
St Peter's Health Centre
Sparkenhoe Street
Leicester LE2 0TA

Tel: 0116 262 5162
Fax: 0116 253 1861

Written or telephone enquiries.

Share Out (Seeking Health Advice, Reassurance and Education Open to Under 20s), Louth, Alford, Mablethorpe and Horncastle

■ Setting
Rural. Health centres and youth centres.

■ Principal aims and objectives
To provide professional guidance, advice and support on a range of health-related issues for young people under 20 and to offer appropriate intervention where needed, sympathetically and non-judgementally, in a confidential, welcoming and accessible setting in rural areas. To provide services complementary to GPs' surgeries and family planning clinics. To reduce the number of unwanted pregnancies in teenagers. To prevent STDs (including HIV) among young people aged 12–20. To improve the emotional and physical well-being of young people by education, information and support to reduce risk-taking behaviour and increase responsible choices towards a healthy lifestyle.

■ Services offered
Staffing. At Louth: 1 physician, 2 nurses (1 school nurse is also counselling trained), 1 male health visitor specialist in sexual health, 1 receptionist/clerk. At outlying sessions: a minimum of 1 physician, 1 nurse, 1 receptionist/clerk.

Advice/counselling. Offered by nurse initially and doctor subsequently if necessary. Referral to child psychiatry/psychology services if required. Pre- and post-termination of pregnancy counselling provided by specialist counsellor at dedicated clinic in Lincoln, but Share Out staff also able to provide this. HIV support by male health visitor, with referral to GUM services as necessary.

Contraception/sexual-health services. Wide range of contraceptives including variety of condoms, strong condoms, lubricant, female condoms, and after-sex emergency contraception. On-the-spot pregnancy testing. Referral for termination of pregnancy. Smear tests. HIV and other STD tests referred to GUM services at Louth.

Tea Shop in Louth town centre staffed by voluntary youth workers from youth service. Share Out staff participate on an informal basis; other services (e.g. legal advice and CAB-type service) being developed.

Open at various times throughout the week, including Friday and Saturday nights.

Health visitor developing work with young men, including sessions in schools.

Telephone line to central clinic provides information on clinic opening times.

■ Appropriateness and accessibility
Services advertised by posters and information cards in schools, libraries and GPs' surgeries.

Occasional articles in local paper.

Share Out venues in towns and villages – two health centres, one youth centre and one voluntary youth project. Additional services at the Tea Shop.

Offer drop-in sessions two lunchtimes in Louth, Saturday late morning in Horncastle, one evening in Mablethorpe and alternate Friday lunchtimes in Alford (term time only).

Lunchtime clinics near secondary schools because of transport difficulties in rural areas.

Signposting; easy access to premises.

Drinks available in some centres.

Health promotion displays.

Confidentiality discussed at first visit. Written policies on confidentiality. Staff trained on confidentiality issues.

Close links with GUM services, schools, youth services (statutory and voluntary), children's homes, community projects and GPs.

■ Evaluation
Monitoring and occasional customer satisfaction surveys. Korner plus greater detail.

■ Contact
Dr Greta Ross
Senior Clinical Medical Officer,
  Child Health
Queen Street Clinic, Queen Street
Louth, Lincolnshire LN11 9BH

Tel: 01507 602568
Fax: 01507 609290

Written or telephone enquiries. Visits by arrangement.

Teenage Information Clinics and Teenage Sexual Health Clinic, Newark, Warsop, Kirkby, Sutton, Ollerton and Mansfield

■ Setting
Towns in rural areas. Health centres.

■ Principal aims and objectives
To provide confidential, non-judgemental advice to all teenagers.

To provide contraceptive advice and care, including information on safer sex and other issues.

■ Services offered
Staffing. 1 physician and 2 nurses at most clinic sessions. In smaller facilities 1 nurse. At town clinic, 1 youth worker for three-month pilot.

Advice/counselling. Provided by nurse and doctor. Developing links with local Youth Information Shop.

Contraception/sexual-health services. Wide range of contraceptives including condoms, strong condoms, lubricant, after-sex emergency contraception. On-the-spot pregnancy testing. Referral for termination of pregnancy. Smear and chlamydia tests. Tests for HIV and other STDs referred to GUM services.

Some work undertaken in schools.

■ Appropriateness and accessibility
Posters and leaflets to schools, youth workers, GPs, libraries and Citizens' Advice Bureaux. Feature article in local newspaper.

Clinics located in local health centres.

Sessions five days a week. Five late afternoon sessions and one midday session.

Music and videos during sessions. Health promotion leaflets and information.

Confidentiality discussed at first visit.

Links with youth service, GUM services, school nurses, social services, child protection team and child health department.

Involved in multi-agency group.

■ Evaluation
Audits on notes and referrals. Korner.

■ **Contact**
Dr Liz Butler
Senior Clinical Medical Officer,
  Family Planning Department
Banks Ward
Mansfield Community Hospital
Stockwell Gate
Mansfield NG18 5QJ

Tel: 01623 785050
Fax: 01623 424062

Written or telephone enquiries.

Victoria Teenage Clinic, Nottingham

■ **Setting**
Urban. Health centre.

■ **Principal aims and objectives**
To provide contraception and general health advice, including pregnancy counselling and help with emotional problems, for any young person.

■ **Services offered**
Staffing. 2 physicians, 3–4 nurses, 1 clinical psychologist (and trainee usually), 2 receptionists/clerks.

Advice/counselling. Sexual-health advice by doctor/nurses. One doctor provides advice on psychosexual matters. Clinical psychologist provides ongoing therapeutic work.

Contraception/sexual-health services. Wide range, including strong condoms and dual method. On-the-spot pregnancy tests. Referral for termination of pregnancy. After-sex emergency contraception. Smear tests.

Six-month trial of chlamydia testing for young people aged 13–19. Referral to GUM services for HIV-related counselling and testing, and testing for other STDs.

Work in schools, youth clubs and other agencies.

Talking About Sex and Pregnancy – 24-hour recorded telephone information line offering advice on contraception, pregnancy and abortion.

■ **Appropriateness and accessibility**
Service promoted by posters and leaflets to health centres, libraries, schools youth clubs and leisure centres.

Consultations on drop-in basis or by appointment.

City centre location, behind shopping centre and bus station.

Follow BMA guidelines on confidentiality. Discuss this with each young person at first visit and advertise it well.

Good links with community paediatrician, police surgeons, homelessness team, children's homes, schools and Parentline. Involved in range of multi-disciplinary forums.

■ **Evaluation**
In-house data collection system, related to method of contraception. Occasional snapshots and user surveys.

■ **Contact**
Dr Ann Howard/ Christine
  Humphries
Consultant Community
  Paediatrician/Clinic Nurse
  Coordinator
Victoria Health Centre
Glasshouse Street
Nottingham
NG1 3LW

Tel: 0115 948 0500
Fax: 0115 941 3371

Telephone or written enquiries.

Sheffield Youth Clinic

■ Setting
City centre. Central clinic.

■ Principal aims and objectives
To provide an accessible, appropriate contraceptive service for young people under 20. To reduce teenage pregnancy, encourage safer sex and prevent HIV and other sexually transmitted diseases. To gain the confidence of young people by providing a confidential service.

■ Services offered
Staffing. 2 physicians, 2–3 nurses, 1 receptionist/clerk, 1 youth worker once a fortnight.

Advice/counselling. Doctor/nurse and youth worker, with referral to youth advice service and to social worker in adolescent unit.

Contraception/sexual health services. Wide range, including strong condoms, female condoms, lubricant. On-the-spot pregnancy testing. Referral for termination of pregnancy. Referral to GUM for HIV counselling and testing.

Outreach by nurses in schools, youth clubs, training schemes.

Training of school nurses in family planning.

■ Appropriateness and accessibility
Centrally located.

Four late afternoon drop-in clinics each week, plus two satellite clinics in local areas.

Television/video during clinic to help with confidentiality.

Work closely with Sheffield Centre for HIV and Sexual Health which supports distribution of posters, leaflets to GPs, youth service.

Young people's phoneline.

Clear and well publicised confidentiality procedures.

■ Evaluation
Audit of condom use, pregnancy rate. Korner.

■ Contact
Anne Ward
Team Leader, Youth Clinic
Central Health Clinic
Mulberry Street
Sheffield S1 1PJ

Tel: 0114 2716790

Written enquiries preferred.

WEST MIDLANDS

Birmingham Brook Advisory Centre, Birmingham

■ Setting
Urban. Dedicated advisory service.

■ Principal aims and objectives
To prevent and mitigate the suffering caused by unintended pregnancy by educating young people about sex and contraception. To develop a sense of responsibility amongst young people with regard to sexual behaviour.

■ Services offered
Staffing. 1 physician, 1 nurse, 1 sessional counsellor, 1 receptionist.

Advice/counselling. Sessional counsellor registers all new users to identify their needs and introduce them to the centre. Crisis counselling, longer-term counselling and psychosexual counselling available.

Contraception/sexual-health services. Wide range including condoms (extra-strong available), cap/diaphragm, after-sex emergency contraception. Smear tests. Pregnancy testing and pregnancy counselling.

Above services offered in four centres – Edgbaston, Birmingham city centre, Handsworth and Saltley.

Outreach work in local community, including schools. Speakers' team gives talks to range of groups and organisations. Sexuality awareness training for teachers, youth workers and school nurses.

Information Shop run jointly with youth services. Basic contraceptive services provided.

Resource Base to be used for group work. Men-only session should start early in 1996.

■ Appropriateness and acceptability
Service advertised by flyers and leaflets. Grant from district health authorities to advertise on buses and billboards.

Consultations on drop-in and appointment basis. Drop-in service for condoms.

Located on good bus route.

Written confidentiality policy is explained to young people when first attending.

Links with education and youth service. Visits to schools, youth groups and voluntary organisations. Members of district health authority forums for young people.

Starter pack containing three condoms distributed with information about Brook.

■ Evaluation
Monitoring of service use and service users (number of contacts, gender, ethnicity). Complaints procedure and suggestions boxes.

■ Contact
Jenny Smith
Director, Client Services
Birmingham Brook Advisory Centre
9 York Road
Edgbaston
Birmingham B16 9HX

Tel: 0121 455 0491
Fax: 0121 454 9474

Written or telephone enquiries.
Visits by arrangement only.

Just for You, Chelmsley Wood, Kingshurst and Solihull

■ Setting
Urban/suburban. Health centres.

Principal aims and objectives
To reduce unintended pregnancies
by providing an acceptable, accessible
and comprehensive contraceptive
service for young men and women
under 20 in Solihull. To provide health
advice, information and counselling.
To raise young people's self-esteem
through individual and group work.
To promote health through peer
dissemination.

■ Services offered
Staffing. 1 physician, 1 nurse, 1 health
education officer, 1 receptionist.

Advice/counselling. One-off counselling
by doctor or nurse. Referral for
ongoing counselling.

Contraception/sexual-health services.
Wide range including condoms,
cap/diaphragm, after-sex emergency
contraception. Smear tests. On-the-
spot pregnancy testing. Referral for
termination of pregnancy.

Work in local schools.

■ Appropriateness and acceptability
Service advertised in schools, youth
clubs, GPs' surgeries, hospitals and
libraries via leaflets. Advertisements
on buses.

Drop-in on Monday, Wednesday and
Thursday late afternoon/early evening
(three different locations).

Disabled access.

Drinks available.

Written confidentiality policy. Each
young person welcomed by health
education officer when first attending
and confidentiality discussed during
an induction session.

Links with youth service, education,
nurse coordinator and local voluntary
organisations. Involved in action topic
groups (e.g. Health of the Nation
groups and young people's multi-
agency strategic group).

■ Evaluation
Korner.

■ Contact
Jo Smith/Michelle Diaz
HIV Coordinator/Health Education
  Officer
Solihull Health Education Services
Solihull Healthcare
20 Union Road
Solihill, Birmingham B91 3EF

Tel: 0121 711 7171
Fax: 0121 704 0341

Trish Embley
Sexual Health and Contraception
  Services Manager
Solihull Healthcare
Craig Croft Clinic
Craig Croft
Chelmsley Wood
Birmingham B37 7TR

Tel: 0121 770 4432

Written enquiries preferred.

Saturday Young People's Clinic, Hereford

■ Setting
Suburban with rural catchment. Health centre.

■ Principal aims and objectives
To promote good sexual health and to reduce pregnancies amongst young people. To offer advice and counselling on relationships and dieting.

■ Services offered
Staffing. 1 physician, 1 nurse, 1 youth adviser/youth worker, 1 receptionist. Rota of young people who sit in the waiting area and welcome other young people to the clinic.

Advice/counselling. Provided by doctor as necessary, with ongoing support. Trained counsellor occasionally available.

Contraception/sexual-health services. Wide range including condoms, cap/diaphragm and after-sex emergency contraception. Smear tests. On-the-spot pregnancy testing. Referral for termination of pregnancy.

Rural Outreach Project for young people aged 16–25. Workers contact young people unable to reach clinic. Leaflets and condoms distributed.

24-hour recorded answering service providing information and opening times of drop-in service.

■ Appropriateness and acceptability
Service advertised via posters and leaflets in schools and youth groups. Stickers in pubs and public lavatories. Also advertised through outreach service.

Service open Saturdays late morning to early afternoon on drop-in basis. Map on all printed publicity. Poster outside clinic on Saturday.

Confidentiality policy advertised on all publicity and emphasised during work in schools and youth groups.

Links with schools, youth service and GUM services.

Training provided to school nurses and teachers. Sessions run for young people in schools and youth groups addressing range of sexual- and drug-related health issues.

■ Evaluation
Monitoring of numbers and ages of young people and area of residence. Note how young people heard of the service and what they felt about it. Report produced every three months. Korner.

■ Contact
Jo Jones
Senior Health Promotion Officer,
  HIV/AIDS and Sexual Health
Herefordshire Health Promotion
Victoria House
Eign Street
Hereford HR4 0AN

Tel: 01432 272012
Fax: 01432 341958

Written or telephone enquiries.

Young People's Clinic, Longbridge

■ Setting
Urban.

Principal aims and objectives
To improve the sexual health of young people in the Longbridge area. To help particularly those under 16. To provide a family planning service

with advice and information in an accessible way to young people.

■ Services offered
Staffing. 1 doctor, 1 nurse, 1 receptionist.

Advice/counselling. Doctor provides pyschosexual counselling and pre- and post-termination of pregnancy counselling. Referrals to voluntary agencies for other counselling.

Outreach. Safer-sex roadshow operates in schools and at open evenings. Talks provided by doctor and health promotion officer.

Contraception/sexual-health services. Oral contraceptives, condoms (including extra-strong and lubricants), dental dams, cap/diaphragm, after-sex emergency contraception. Smears. On-the-spot pregnancy testing. Referral for termination of pregnancy.

■ Appropriateness and accessibility
Service advertised via cards, leaflets, posters distributed in schools, libraries, youth services, colleges, GPs' surgeries and youth clubs. Adverts on buses.

Service open Monday late afternoon/early evening. Near bus route. Refreshments available. Music and television. Drop-in only.

Written code of confidentiality stated on all advertising. Young people informed of policy by receptionist.

Links with the youth service, primary care teams, schools and marginalised young people.

■ Evaluation
Written ten-month review which informs service development. Korner.

■ Contact
Lucy Loveless
Health Promotion Division
St Patricks Centre
  for Community Health
Highgate Street
Birmingham B12 0YA

Tel: 0121 446 4747
Fax: 0121 445 6596

Telephone enquiry preferred.

The Health Store, Nuneaton

■ Setting
Suburban. Youth centre.

■ Principal aims and objectives
To provide a client-led, holistic health and welfare service which responds to the needs of young people in north Warwickshire. To not only provide contraception services but also respond to other health and welfare needs.

■ Services offered
Staffing. 1 doctor, 1 nurse, 2 sessional counsellors, 1 health promotion officer, 1 receptionist.

Advice/counselling. Crisis counselling, pre- and post-termination of pregnancy counselling, relationship and some ongoing counselling. Referrals to child psychology service via GP.

Contraception/sexual-health services. Oral contraception, condoms (some extra strong), cap/diaphragm, after-sex emergency contraception service. Smears. On-the-spot pregnancy testing, referral for abortion. All clinical testing referred to GUM services.

Outreach. Weekly session at local college, provision of pregnancy testing

and some contraceptives (not pill).
Other outreach to leaving-care group;
careers department; young lesbian, gay
and bisexual group; young mothers.
24-hour recorded message service.

Library for young people, with access
to health promotion resources.

■ Appropriateness and accessibility

Service advertised by leaflets and
posters via schools, youth centres,
GPs' surgeries, social services, health
promotion services and family
planning clinics. Features in local
free papers. Visit to centre part of
induction of Trust staff.

Service open at varying times (not
Wednesdays or Fridays). Outreach
to local college one day per week,
group work at other times. Centre
2–3 minutes' walk from town centre.
Appointments and drop-in service.

Based in youth centre. Dedicated
space for young people's health needs.

Clear confidentiality policy. Written
policy displayed in centre.
Confidentiality statement on all
publicity.

Close links with range of agencies
including health promotion,
alcohol/drugs advisory service, social
services, local college and schools.

■ Evaluation

Feedback sheets. Monitoring of
number of young people using service.
Six-monthly reports. Korner.

■ Contact

Liz Biolik
Health Promotion Specialist, Project
  Coordinator of Health Store
Hatter's Space
Upper Abbey Street
Nuneaton CV11 5DH

Tel: 01203 351418
Fax: 01203 351434
(mark f.a.o. Liz Biolik)

Written or telephone enquiries.
Visits by arrangement.

Sexual Health Drop-in, Oldbury

■ Setting

Urban. Health centre.

■ Principal aims and objectives

To provide advice, information and
free condoms to young people. To
act as a referral agency and, where
needed, to accompany young people
using other services. To provide
ongoing support to people living with,
and affected by, HIV and AIDS. To
provide health promotion services.

■ Services offered

Staffing. 1 nurse, 1 outreach worker
(for men who have sex with men),
1 HIV counsellor, no administrative
support at present. 1 sexual-health
development worker to work with
African-Caribbean young people.

Advice/counselling. Provide advice
about contraception. Recorded out-
of-hours answering machine message
about HIV, family planning services
and emergency contraception.
Advice/counselling for people living
with, and affected by, HIV and AIDS.

Contraception/sexual-health services.
Range of condoms, female condoms
and other safer sex resources
including dental dams. Correct
condom use demonstrated with every
new client. Referrals for emergency
contraception.

Training in sexual health undertaken
with professional groups such as
teachers, youth workers and social

workers. Training also provided to school governors.

Support to GPs and voluntary organis-ations provided via pilot Community Condoms Project, whereby condoms are sensitively made available to young people via primary health-care teams and voluntary organisations.

Roadshows for young homeless people and youth training organisations.

Saturday afternoon Young Person's Clinic.

■ Appropriateness and acceptability
Service advertised in specially produced youth magazines (young people involved in design and production) and at youth clubs, via posters, newspapers, radio and using a telephone information line.

Service open Monday late afternoon/early evening and by appointment at other times.

Near to the station.

Confidentiality policy. Training and education provided to staff on confidentiality matters.

Links with Sexual Health Commis-sioning Group, local schools and youth groups, Brook Advisory Service.

■ Evaluation
Monitoring of gender and ethnicity of young people using service.

■ Contact
Sarah New/Dr I Blair
Specialist Nurse
Unity Centre
6 Unity Place
Oldbury B69 4DB

Tel: 0121 544 3737
Fax: 0121 544 2094

Written or telephone enquiries.

Teen Clinic and Drop-in Clinic, Tipton

■ Setting
Multi-ethnic inner city area. GP/health centre.

■ Principal aims and objectives
Teen Clinic: to provide a health promotion service to young people around their 16th birthday, which includes advice on sexual health, drug and substance use, and other health issues.

Drop-in Clinic: to promote the sexual health of young people through on-the-spot advice on sexual health and other health matters.

■ Services offered
Staffing. 1 or more doctors, 1 school nurse, 1 health visitor.

Advice/counselling. Provided through the Teen Clinic on a range of health matters. Crisis counselling, counselling for after-sex emergency contraception, and counselling/advice for other health problems provided through the Drop-in Clinic.

Contraception/sexual-health services. Large range of condoms (including extra-strong) and other contraceptive services. On-the-spot pregnancy testing. After-sex emergency contraception, including special card to be handed to clinic receptionist for urgent appointment. Referrals for other services.

Work with local schools by school nurse attached to clinic.

■ Appropriateness and accessibility
Teen Clinic promoted via personal invitation on 16th birthday to young people registered with the practice.

Drop-in Clinic promoted via posters/flyers in local schools and in surgery/health centre.

Services provided one day a week after school hours.

Service provided in general use clinic room with own entrance adjacent to health centre.

Both services aim to adhere to principles of confidentiality, trust, reliability, approachability and accessibility.

■ **Evaluation**
Currently monitor number and age of clinic attenders, and number of condoms distributed. Further evaluation planned.

■ **Contact**
Dr Tony Robinson
Black Country Family Practice Health
  Centre
Queens Road
Tipton DY4 8PH

Tel: 0121 557 6397
Fax: 0121 557 1662

Contact by letter or telephone.

Young Person's Clinic, West Bromwich

■ **Setting**
Urban. Health centre.

■ **Principal aims and objectives**
To achieve the Health of the Nation targets in relation to unintended pregnancy. To reduce local rates of unintended pregnancy by 50 per cent by the year 2000.

Services offered
Staffing. 1 doctor, 2 nurses, 2 receptionists.

Advice/counselling. Provided by doctor and nurse. Information/advice telephone line covered by family planning nurses at weekdays.

Contraception/sexual-health services. Include oral contraception, condoms (extra-strong available), cap/diaphragm, after-sex emergency contraception. Smear tests. On-the-spot pregnancy testing. Referral for termination of pregnancy.

Clinical testing. Referral to GUM services, which can provide pre- and post-test HIV counselling.

■ **Appropriateness and accessibility**
Service advertised via flyers and posters to all school nurses. Some newspaper and radio advertising at start of project.

Central location opposite bus station. Consultation on drop-in and appointment basis. Service offered on Saturday afternoon. Music.

Explicit statement of confidentiality on all promotional literature. Sessions in schools to inform young people of confidentiality procedure.

Links with service for young women with unintended pregnancy.

■ **Evaluation**
Audit of views of young people aged under 16 to identify their perceptions of sex education. Korner.

■ **Contact**
Jean Foster
Senior Sister, Family Planning
Cronehills Health Centre
Cronehill Linkway
West Bromwich

Tel: 0121 553 1316

Telephone or written enquiries.

BIBLIOGRAPHY

Abdullah, S. (1993) 'GPs, teenagers and sex', *British Journal of Sexual Medicine*. vol. 20, no. 2, pp. 13–14.

Allaby, M. (1995) 'Contraceptive services for teenagers: do we need family planning services?', *British Medical Journal*. no. 310, pp. 1641–3.

Allen, I. (1991) *Family planning and pregnancy counselling projects for young people*. Policy Studies Institute Publishing, London.

Brook Advisory Centres (1994) *Private and confidential: talking to doctors*. Brook Advisory Centres, London.

Carlin, E. M., Russell, J. M., Sibley, K. & Boag, F. C. (1995) 'Evaluating a designated family planning clinic within a genitourinary medicine service', *Genitourinary Medicine*. vol. 71, pp. 106–8.

Committee on Child Health Services (1976) *Fit for the future* [the Court Report]. HMSO, London.

Cooper, P., Diamond, I., High, S. & Pearson, S. (1994) 'A comparison of family planning provision: general practice and family planning clinics', *British Journal of Family Planning*. vol. 19, pp. 263–9.

Davidson, N. & Lloyd, T. (1993) *Working with heterosexual men on sexual health*. Health Education Authority, London.

Department of Health and Social Security (1984) *Family planning and abortion services for young people*. HC (84) 34. London.

Department of Health and Social Security (1988) *Health services development*. HC (88) 43. London.

Department of Health (1993) *Key area handbook HIV/AIDS and sexual health*. Department of Health, Heywood, Lancs.

Department of Health (1994) *One year on*. Department of Health, Heywood, Lancs.

Elias, C. & Leonard, A. (1995) 'Family planning and sexually transmitted diseases: the need to enhance contraceptive choice', *Current Issues in Public Health*. vol. 1, pp. 191-9.

Family Planning Association (1990) *Family planning services: a model for health authorities*. Family Planning Association, London.

Family Planning Association (1992) *The legal position regarding contraceptive advice and provision to young people*. FPA factsheet. Family Planning Association, London.

Fleissig, A. (1992) 'Family planning services – use and preferences of recent mothers', *British Journal of Family Planning*. vol. 17, pp. 110–14.

HEA (1992) *Today's young people*. Health Education Authority, London.

Jewitt, C. (1995) *Brook and men evaluation report: developing young men's sexual health initiatives*. Health First, London.

Kirkpatrick, J. (1994) 'Are young people using sexual health services?', *Youth Clubs*. September, pp. 16–19.

McAvoy, B. R. (1985) 'Communication skills and family planning doctors', *British Journal of Family Planning*. vol. 11, 44–9.

Masters, L., Nicholas, H., Bunting, P. & Welch, J. (1995) 'Family planning in genitourinary medicine: an opportunistic service?', *Genitourinary Medicine*. vol. 71, 103–5.

NHS Management Executive (1992) *Guidelines for reviewing family planning services: guidance for regions*. NHSME, London.

Packham, S. (1993) 'Streetwise but clinic shy', *Nursing Standard*. vol. 13, vol. 8, pp. 18–19.

Peach, E., Harris, J. & Bielby, E. (1994) *Teenage pregnancy – a community issue*. A report by the Yorkshire Collaborating Centre for Health Services Research. University of Leeds, Nuffield Institute for Health, Leeds.

Peckham, S. (1993) 'Preventing unintended teenage pregnancies', *Public Health*. vol. 107, pp. 125–33.

Phillips, D. (1992) 'Changing sexual lifestyles of young people: implications for family planning', in Royal College of General Practitioners, *1992 members' reference book*. RCGP, London.

Podmore, J. (1992) 'The future of family planning services in the UK', *British Journal of Sexual Medicine*. January/February, pp. 18–21.

Royal College of Obstetricians and Gynaecologists (1991) *Report of the RCOG working party on unplanned pregnancy*. London.

Scally, G. & Hadley, A. (1995) 'Accessibility of sexual health services for young people: survey of clinics in a region', *Journal of Management in Medicine*. vol. 9, vol. 4, pp. 51–2.

Scott, J. (1994) *Family planning services in Suffolk: report of a consultation with under 16 year-olds in Suffolk*. Suffolk Health Authority/Suffolk Family Health Services Authority, Ipswich.

Scott, J. (1995) 'School's out ... for family planning', *Nursing Standard*. vol. 9, no. 45, 20–1.

Stedman, Y. & Elstein, M. (1995) 'Rethinking sexual health clinics', *British Medical Journal*. vol. 310, pp. 342–3.

Strauss, G. (1992) 'Not for the boys', *AIDS Dialogue*. no. 17.

Thin, R. N., Whatley, J. D. & Smith, C. (1989) 'STD and contraception in adolescents', *Genitourinary Medicine*. vol. 65, 157–60.

Thompson, E. & Chapple, J. (1994) 'Taking a bearing – a regional perspective of family planning provision', *British Journal of Family Planning*. vol. 19, 278–81.

United Nations (1994) *Programme of action of the United Nations International Conference on Population and Development*. United Nations, New York.

Walling, M. (1995) 'The TAC-1 project', *British Journal of Sexual Medicine*. July/August, pp. 30–1.

Ward, H., Kubba, A., Bradbeer, C., Pillaye, J. & Randall, S. (1995) *Report from consensus workshop on sexually transmitted diseases and contraception: sexual health promotion and service delivery*. Faculty of Family Planning and Reproductive Health Care/Faculty of Public Health Medicine/Medical Society for the Study of Venereal Diseases, London.

Wardle, S. & Wright, P. (1993) 'Family planning services – the needs of young people', *British Journal of Family Planning*. vol. 19, 158–60.

West, J., Hudson, F., Levitas, R. & Guy, W. (1995) *Young people and clinics: providing for sexual health in Avon*. University of Bristol, Department of Sociology, Bristol.

Wilson, S. & Heslop, C. (1991) 'Do we need local family planning clinics?', *British Journal of Family Planning*. vol. 17, pp. 49–52.

Wilson, S. (1993) 'Services to promote the sexual health of young people', in Working Group of the Department of Public Health Medicine and Epidemiology, *Promoting the sexual health of young people*. University Hospital Queens Medical Centre, Nottingham.

Wilson, S., Denman, S., Gillies, P. & Wijewardene, K. (1994) 'Purchasing services to promote the sexual health of young people – contraceptive care for teenagers', *European Journal of Public Health*. vol. 4, pp. 207–12.

INDEX

Most of the centres offer a wide range of services. Therefore, if a particular service is required (e.g. smear test, pregnancy test, contraception provision/advice) it is suggested that the reader looks up a particular clinic/centre or location to check availability.

Abrahams, *Dr* Jackie 51
acceptability of service: monitoring
      see monitoring of services access to
            services 3, 4
Adolescent Clinics, Ripon 24
advertising of services 4
advice/counselling 4
      see also psychosexual counselling
      crisis counselling 5
      HIV-related counselling 4
      services offered *see* individual
            clinic/centre entries
Advisory Centre for Young People,
      Salisbury 43
after-sex emergency contraception 3
'agony aunt' columns 13
Alford: Share Out 53–4
Allen, *Dr* Pauline 40
Alnwick: The Pop Inn 18–19
Always, Doncaster 50–1
Anglia and Oxford region:
            clinics/centres 11–17
approachability of staff 5
appropriateness of service: monitoring
      see monitoring of services
arcades: services near/in
      see location of services
assessments of needs: monitoring
      see monitoring of services
atmosphere of centre/clinic 4–5
attitudes of staff 5

Barking: Young Person's Health Advice
      Service 30–1
Barnett, Margaret 22
Batchelor, *Dr* Lesley 36
Bean, *Dr* Brenda 26
Bexleyheath:
      Youth Advisory Clinic 44
Biolik, Liz 61
Birkenhead: Wirral Brook Advisory
      Centre 32
Birmingham Brook Advisory
      Centre 57–8
Blackfen:
      Youth Advisory Clinic 44
Blair, *Dr* I. 62
Bodywise, Kettering 12–13
Bolton:
      Teenage Advisory Clinic 33
Booth, Liz 24
Bournemouth: The Junction
      Health Advisory Centre 38
Bowden, Karen 28
Brighton: Young People's Drop-in
      Clinic 45
Brook Advisory Centre
      Birmingham 57–8
      Cornwall 42–3
      London 28, 47–8
      Merseyside 34–5
      Wirral 32
Brown, Lori 13
Burgess, Gina 31

Burnham-on-Sea: Young Adults'
      Drop-in Clinic 38–9
Bury St Edmunds:
      Walk-In Clinic 11
Butler, *Dr* Liz 55

Carlisle: Youth Counselling
        Service/Raffles Counselling
        Service 19
characteristics of services: of listed
        centres/clinics 6–7
Chatham:
        Young Person's Clinic 46
Chelmsley Wood: Just for You 58
Chichester: Sussed Sex,
        'Number 18' 46–7
Children Act Assessments: advocacy
        service 14
chlamydia tests
        Bolton 33
        Gateshead 20
        Ilkeston 51
        Nottinghamshire 54, 55
        South Shields 25
Choices, Doncaster 50–1
City and Hackney Young People's
        Services, London 26–7
clothes: of staff 5
Coleford Health Centre,
        Gloucester 39–40
colleges: services near/in
        see location of services
communication skills 5
community-based outreach
        work 3, 6–7^t
Community Clinic for Young People,
        Southampton/Shirley/New
        Milton/Romsey/Thornhill 40–1
Community Information System 12
concerts 40
condoms 3
        see also individual clinic/centre
        entries
        Denton 33
        Ilkeston 51
        Leicester 52
        Liverpool 35
        London 27, 28
        Longbridge 59
        Newcastle upon Tyne 23
        Sheffield 56
confidentiality 5

contraception
        see also individual clinic/centre
        entries
        provision/advice 3, 4
Cornwall Brook Advisory Centre,
        Redruth 42–3
counselling
        see advice/counselling
County Council Information Terminal,
        Oxford 16
Cozens, Janet 51
crisis counselling 57
Curtis, Kay 17

decoration of waiting areas 4
Denton: Tameside Young People's
        Health Clinic/Peer Education
        Project 33–4
Deptford: Liaison 47–8
Derby: Under 20s Clinic/Free
        Condom Clinics 49
Designated Young People's Clinics,
        Leeds 21-2
developing a service 3-8
Diaz, Michelle 58
disabled access 4
disabled people 5
Doncaster: Choices/Youth
        Clinic/Always 50-1
Douglas, Pam 23
Drink Sense 17
Drop-in Clinic, Tipton 62–3
DSS support 14
dual methods of contraception 3
Duke Street Clinic,
        Denton 33–4

Edgbaston: Birmingham Brook
        Advisory Centre 57
effects of service provision:
        evaluating 5
Ellis, Dr Sylvia 47
Embley, Trish 58
emergency contraception 3
equal opportunities 5
Erith: Youth Advisory Clinic 44

ethnic communities 5
evaluation of services 5, 11, 23, 50–1
extra-strong condoms 3

Family Planning Clinics,
      Peterborough 16–17
Family Planning Services
   London 47–8
   Oxford 15–16
   Queensway Health Centre,
      Hatfield 26
female condoms 3
Foster, Jean 63
Francis, Glynnis 34
Free Condom Clinics, Derby 49

Gaffney, Justin 29
Gallagher, *Dr* Janet 25
Gateshead:
      Young Person's Clinic 19–20
gay men 5
Gay Men's Health Project 14
general health services 4
General Practitioner (GP)
      practices 3, 6–7[t]
   advertising of services 4
Gloucester: Healthwise,
      Coleford Health Centre 39–40
GPs *see* General Practitioner
      (GP) practices
Grapevine, The, South Shields 25
Greenhall, *Dr* Liz 16
Gurr, Rosalie 41

Hall, Liz 35
Hampton: Community Clinic for
      Young People 40–1
Handsworth: Birmingham Brook
      Advisory Centre 57
Harrow:
      Young People's Service 29–30
Hatfield:
      Family Planning Service,
      Queensway Health Centre 26
Haverhill:
      Young Person's Clinic 11

health-day displays 11
health fairs 40
Health Information Shop 14
Health Rave 24
health services 4
Health Store, The, Nuneaton 60–1
Healthwise, Coleford Health Centre,
      Gloucester 39–40
Healthy Alliance Award 31
Heathcote, Gill 27
Hellon, June 19
helplines, telephone *see* telephone
      helplines/information lines
Hereford: Saturday Young People's
      Clinic 59
heterosexual men 5
Hexham Young People's Clinic 20–1
HIV (human immunodeficiency
      virus)
   HIV-related counselling 4
   prevention/treatment 4
Holt, Lesley 20
Horncastle: Share Out 53–4
Howard, *Dr* Ann 55
Hoyle, Liz 19
human immunodeficiency virus
      see HIV
Humphries, Christine 56
Huntingdon: Newtown Health and
      Advice 11–12

Ilkeston: SHOP (Sexual Health
      Options Project) 51
image of centre/clinic 4–5
information lines
      see telephone helplines/information
      lines
integrated services *see* service
      integration
interpreters 48

Jones, Jo 59
Junction Health Advisory Centre, The,
      Bournemouth 38
Just for You, Chelmsley
      Wood/Kingshurst/Solihull 58

Keep It Safe and Sexy, London
      see KISS
Kettering: Bodywise 12–13
Key area handbook HIV/AIDS and
      sexual health 8
Kingshurst: Just for You 58
Kirkby: Teenage Clinic 54–5
KISS (Keep It Safe and Sexy),
      London Brook Advisory Centre,
      London 28

learning difficulties: people with 5
Leeds
      Designated Young People's
            Clinics 21–2
      The Men's Room 21–2
Leggett, Jeannie 18
Leicester: Young People's Clinic 52–3
lesbians 5
Liaison, Deptford 47–8
Lions Clubs 13
Litton, Heather 39
Liverpool: Merseyside Brook Advisory
      Centre 34–5
local radio: advertising of services 4,
      39, 42
location of services 4
      near to public transport
            Brighton 45
            Chatham 46
            Liverpool 34
            London 27, 28
            Newcastle upon Tyne 23
            Romford/Barking 30
            South Shields 25
            Warrington 37
      near to/in colleges
            Brighton 45
            Kettering 13
            Romford/Barking 30
            Warrington 36
      near to/in meeting places
            Chelmsley Wood/Kingshurst/
                  Solihull 58
            Oldbury 61
            West Bromwich 63

location of services (contd.)
      near to/in schools
            Alnwick 18
            Carlisle 19
            Chelmsley Wood/Kingshurst/
                  Solihull 58
            Denton 34
            Leeds 22
            Lincolnshire 53
            New Milton/Romsey/
                  Thornhill 40
            Romford/Barking 30
            Warrington 36
            West Bromwich 63
      near to/in shopping centres
            Birkenhead 32
            Birmingham 57
            Merseyside 34
            Newcastle upon Tyne 23
      near to/in youth centres
            Birmingham 57
            Bournemouth 38
            Chelmsley Wood/Kingshurst/
                  Solihull 58
            Chichester 47
            Denton 34
            Doncaster 50
            Hexham 20
            Leicester 52
            Lincolnshire 53
            London 28
            New Milton/Romsey/
                  Thornhill 40
            Norwich 14
            Oldbury 61
            Portsmouth 41
            Redruth 42
            Romford/Barking 30
London
      Brook Advisory Centre 28
      City and Hackney Young
            People's Services 26–7
      Family Planning
            Services 47–8
      Well Men's Service 28–9

Longbridge: Young People's
    Clinic 59–60
Louth: Share Out 53–4
Loveless, Lucy 60

Mablethorpe: Share Out 53–4
Macclesfield: Young People's
    Family Planning Clinic 35–6
magazines: in waiting areas 5, 18,
    30, 62
management committees 14
Mancroft Advice Project, Norwich 14
Mansfield: Teenage Clinic 54–5
men's clinics 4, 6–7[t]
Men's Room, The, Leeds 21–2
Merseyside Brook Advisory Centre,
    Liverpool 34–5
Milchem, Alison 41
Millar, Margaret 24
Milner-Scott, Ruth 43
minority ethnic communities 5
monitoring of services 5
    assessments of needs
        Bexleyheath 44
        Doncaster 50
        Healthwise 40
        Huntingdon 12
        Lincolnshire 54
        Newcastle upon Tyne 23
        Nuneaton 61
    service appropriateness/
        acceptability
        Alnwick 18
        Bexleyheath 44
        Brighton 45
        Chatham 46
        Chichester 47
        Gateshead 19
        Gloucester 40
        Kettering 13
        Leeds 22
        Newcastle upon Tyne 23
        Nuneaton 61
        Oldbury 62
        Portsmouth 42
        Ripon 24
        Romford/Barking 30

    service-user characteristics
        Alnwick 18
        Birkenhead 32
        Birmingham 57
        Brighton 45
        Doncaster 50
        Hereford 59
        Huntingdon 12
        Liverpool 34
        London 28
        Newcastle upon Tyne 23
        Oldbury 62
    music: in waiting areas see waiting
        areas

Nash, Dr Kate 15
needs, assessments of: monitoring
    see monitoring of services
New, Sarah 62
New Milton: Community Clinic for
    Young People 40–1
Newark: Teenage Clinic 54–5
Newcastle upon Tyne:
    Streetwise 22–3
newspapers
    advertising of services 25, 39,
        42, 61
    'agony aunt' columns 13
Newtown Health and Advice,
    Huntingdon 11–12
Noden, Judi 33
'non-judgemental' attitudes 5
'non-traditional' service users 5
North Thames region:
    clinics/centres 26–31
North West Anglia Health Care
    Trust 17
Northern and Yorkshire region:
    clinics/centres 18–25
North West region:
    clinics/centres 32–7
Northwick Park Hospital 30
Norwich
    Mancroft Advice Project 14
    Young Person's Clinic/Under 25s
        Clinic 14–15

Nottingham: Victoria Teenage
    Clinic 55–6
'Number 18' (Sussed Sex),
    Chichester 46–7
Nuneaton: The Health Store 60–1

Oldbury: Sexual Health Drop-in 61–2
Ollerton: Teenage Clinic 54–5
on-the-spot pregnancy tests 3
on-the-spot STD tests 4
opening times 4
Optimum Health Services,
    London 47–8
outreach work 3, 6–7[t]
Owen-Smith, *Dr* Angela 12
Oxford:
    Family Planning Services 15–16
Oxford and Anglia region:
    clinics/centres 11–17

Palmer, Pat 38
Parentline 55
Peer Education Project, Denton 33–4
Percival, Gloria 49
Peterborough: Family Planning and
    Young Person Service – Youth
    Clinics 16–17
Place, The, St Neots 11–12
Plant, Zoe 48
Pop Inn, The, Alnwick 18–19
Portsmouth: Sex Sense 41–2
pregnancy, termination of:
    advice/referral 4
pregnancy tests 3
Prior, Sandy 42
psychosexual counselling
    Birmingham 57
    Chatham 46
    Haverhill/Bury St Edmunds 11
    Leicester 52
    London 47
    Longbridge 60
    Nottingham 55
    Oxford 15
public transport: services near *see*
    location of services

Queensway Health Centre,
    Hatfield 26

radio, local: advertising of services
    4, 39, 42
Raffles Counselling Service,
    Carlisle 19
range of services 3–4
Redruth: Cornwall Brook Advisory
    Centre 42–3
Reed, Dr Bela 30
refreshments: in waiting areas *see*
    waiting areas
Regional Health Information Line,
    Oxford 16
regional listings of clinics/centres
    11–63
Reid, Trish 37
Ripon: Adolescent Clinics/Young
    People's Clinic 24
roadshows 11, 30, 62
Robinson, Ian 23
Robinson, *Dr* Tony 63
Rolph, Justin 14
Romford: Young Person's Health
    Advice Service 30–1
Romsey: Community Clinic for Young
    People 40–1
Ross, Dr Greta 54
Ruddy, Pauline 46
Rural Outreach Project, Hereford 59
Rust, Jean 32
Ryrie, Sue 35

St Neots: The Place 11–12
Salisbury: Advisory Centre for Young
    People 43
Saltley: Birmingham Brook Advisory
    Centre 57
Sanders, Jan 43
Saturday Young People's Clinic,
    Hereford 59
schools: services near/in *see* location
    of services
seating arrangements: in waiting
    areas 5

Seeking Health Advice, Reassurance and Education Open to Under 20s *see* Share Out
selection of staff 5
service characteristics: of listed centres/clinics 6–7t
service integration 4, 6–7t
  Alnwick 18
  Hexham 21
  Kettering 13
  Leeds 22
  Lincolnshire 53
  London 27
  Newcastle upon Tyne 23
  Norwich 14
  Nuneaton 60
  Oldbury 61
  Ripon 24
service settings 3
service-user characteristics: monitoring *see* monitoring of services
services: range of 3–4
setting up a service 3–8
settings of services 3
Sex Action Group 25
sex offenders 13
Sex Sense, Portsmouth 41–2
sexual abuse survivors 14
Sexual Health Drop-in, Oldbury 61–2
Sexual Health Options Project, Ilkeston *see* SHOP
sexual health services 3–4
  see also individual clinic/centre entries
sexually transmitted diseases *see* STD services; STD tests; STDs
Shah, Iram 23
Share Out, Louth/Alford/ Mablethorpe/Horncastle 53–4
Sheffield Centre for HIV and Sexual Health 56
Sheffield Youth Clinic 56
SHOP (Sexual Health Options Project), Ilkeston 51
shopping centres: services near/in *see* location of services

signposting of services 4, 20, 25, 41, 54, 59
smear tests 3
Smith, *Dr* Claire 11
Smith, Jenny 58
Smith, Jo 58
Smith, Tim 34
Solihull: Just for You 58
South and West region: clinics/centres 38–43
South Shields: The Grapevine 25
South Thames region: clinics/centres 44–8
specialist clinics 3, 6–7t
staff
  clothing 5
  selection 5
  training 5, 6–7t
  types *see* individual clinic/centre entries
STD services
  referral to 4
    Huntingdon 11
    Kettering 13
    London 27
    Newcastle upon Tyne 23
    South Shields 25
STD tests 4, 27
STDs (sexually transmitted diseases): prevention/treatment 4
Streetlevel 25
Streetwise, Newcastle upon Tyne 22–3
Suffolk Sexual Health Focus Group 11
summer community concerts 40
Sussed Sex, 'Number 18', Chichester 46–7
Sutton: Teenage Clinic 54–5

Tameside Young People's Health Clinic, Denton 33–4
Teen Clinic, Tipton 62–3
Teenage Advisory Clinic, Bolton 33
Teenage Information Clinics, Nottinghamshire 54–5

Teenage Sexual Health Clinic,
    Nottinghamshire 54–5
telephone helplines/information lines
    Barking 3
    Bolton 33
    Bury St Edmunds 11
    Carlisle 19
    Derby 49
    Hampshire 40
    Haverhill 11
    Hereford 59
    Huntingdon/St Neots 12
    Kettering 13
    Leicester 52
    London 28, 48
    Nottingham 55
    Peterborough 17
    Redruth 42
    Romford 31
    Sheffield 56
television: in waiting areas see waiting
    areas
termination of pregnancy:
    advice/referral 4
tests see chlamydia tests; pregnancy
    tests; STD tests
Thames region: clinics/centres 26–31,
    44-8
Thornhill: Community Clinic for
    Young People 40–1
Tipton: Teen Clinic/Drop-in Clinic
    62–3
trailers 13
training of staff 5, 6-7[t]
Travelling Youth Advice Shop Service,
    Warrington 36
Trent region: clinics/centres 49–56
Turner, Dr Gill 21
Turner, Dr Lynda 20

Under 20s Clinic, Derby 49
Under 25s Clinic, Norwich 14–15

vans/trailers 13
Victoria Teenage Clinic,
    Nottingham 55–6

videos: in waiting areas see waiting
    areas

waiting areas 4–5
    magazines 5, 18, 30, 62
    music
        Alnwick 18
        Bexleyheath 44
        Birkenhead 32
        Chatham 46
        Derby 49
        Hampshire 40
        Harrow 30
        Hexham 20
        Huntingdon 12
        Ilkeston 51
        Newark/Warsop/Kirkby 52
        Newcastle upon Tyne 22
    refreshments
        Alnwick 18
        Chatham 46
        Chelmsley Wood/Kingshurst/
            Solihull 58
        Derby 49
        Gloucester 40
        Hampshire 40
        Hexham 20
        Huntingdon 12
        Ilkeston 51
        Lincolnshire 53
        London 27, 28
        Norwich 14
        Ripon 24
    television
        Alnwick 18
        Newark/Warsop/Kirkby 53
        Oxford 15
        Sheffield 56
    videos
        Alnwick 18
        Gateshead 19
        Hampshire 40
        Huntingdon 12
        Newark/Warsop/Kirkby 53
        Sheffield 56

Walk-In Clinic,
      Bury St Edmunds 11
Walters, Chris 47
Wandless, *Dr* Gill 52
Ward, Anne 56
Ward, Sue 45
Warnock, Cullagh 23
Warrington:
      The Youth Advice Shop 36–7
Warsop: Teenage Clinic 54–5
Well Men's Service, London 28–9
West and South region:
      clinics/centres 38–43
West Bromwich:
      Young Person's Clinic 63
West Midlands:
      clinics/centres 57–63
Willis, Maureen 44
Wirral Brook Advisory Centre,
      Birkenhead 32
Women's Health Information
      Service 14
word of mouth: advertising of
      services 4
World AIDS Day 20, 49

YMCA 45
Yorkshire and Northern region:
      clinics/centres 18–25
Young Adults' Drop-in Clinic,
      Burnham-on-Sea 38–9
Young Carers 13
Young Farmers' groups 42
Young Men's Outreach,
      London 47–8

Young People's Clinic
      Denton 33–4
      Leicester 52–3
      Longbridge 59–60
      Ripon 24
Young People's Drop-in Clinic,
      Brighton 45
Young People's Family Planning
      Clinic, Macclesfield 35–6
young people's forum 14
Young People's Service,
      Harrow 29–30
Young Person Service,
      Peterborough 16–17
Young Person's Clinic
      Chatham 46
      Gateshead 19–20
      Haverhill 11
      Norwich 14–15
      West Bromwich 63
Young Person's Health Advice Service,
      Romford/Barking 30–1
Youth Advice Shop, The,
      Warrington 36–7
Youth Advisory Clinic,
      Bexleyheath/Blackfen/Erith 44
youth advisory services 3, 6–7[t]
youth centres: services near/in *see*
      location of services
Youth Clinic
      Doncaster 50–1
      Peterborough 16–17
Youth Counselling Service,
      Carlisle 19